WHERE THERE IS NO
COSMETIC COUNTER

HOW NOT TO LOOK LIKE A ZOMBIE –
EVEN AFTER THE END OF THE WORLD AS YOU KNOW IT

છ્રછ્રછ્રછ્રછ્રછ્રછ્રછ્રછ્રછ્રછ્રછ્રછ્રછ્રછ્રછ્રછ્રછ્ર

DISCLAIMER

I'm not a cosmetologist or esthetician, although with the money I've spent over the years on cosmetics and beauty products you would think I should have at least been given an honorary certificate of some sort. I am not a beauty consultant either. And I am most definitely not a chemist or a scientist. Plain and simple, I am a woman who does not want to find herself "without" should the proverbial "poo" ever hit-the-fan and, I want to share some of little beauty secrets I've learned along the way made with simple ingredients we have in our home pantries and gardens.

I will however caution you that I have not used all of the suggestions, remedies and treatments you will find in this book. We all are different and what works for one may not always work well for others. These remedies and treatments were written with a scenario in mind where you may no longer have access to your favorite beauty and hygiene products through conventional means due to a number of life changing scenarios. This book is not intended to give medical advice, diagnose, cure, prevent or treat, any disease or skin condition; and should not be used in lieu of seeking medical advice.

I will also caution you to use these remedies and treatments at your own risk as I take no responsibility for their use. If you are unsure about using any of these remedies, treatments, suggestions or a particular item or substance please consult your physician before using. Keep in mind that anything, even natural products and ingredients, can cause an allergy so always spot test!!! In other words, if in doubt, test any substance in question on a small area of your skin first. If any redness, swelling or sensitivity occurs discontinue its use immediately! If you have a severe skin condition you should consult your doctor or dermatologist. Just sayin'.

ॐॐॐॐॐॐॐॐॐॐॐॐॐॐॐॐॐॐॐॐॐॐॐॐॐॐॐॐ

DEDICATION

Some say behind a great man is a great woman. Although it may sound cliché-ish in my situation, it was actually a great man who took the time; and a lot of patience, to explain the world I had only known through the eyes of rose-colored glasses. This new "awakening" prompted me to begin my own journey into disaster survival and preparedness. What I have learned, I now share with others to help promote more awareness for the need to always be prepared. To this man, I will always be truly grateful.

To the other man in my life, thank you for believing in me through the good and the bad.

To my two older sisters (I love saying that) thank you for put up with all the blue eye shadow, pink rouge, red lipstick, and mom's dresses, hats and oversized heels - all in my quest to look "gorgeous".

To my younger brother, thank you for your willingness to act as a stand-in model when the cat was nowhere to be found.

Lastly, thank you Mom and Dad for believing in me and encouraging me to "go-for-it" on whatever I set my sights on. You are both loved and missed so very, very much.

Special thanks to "the doctor".

ରେ ରେ

FORWARD

Knowing how to maintain a sense of well-being and hygiene in an end of our world as we know it scenario - where we no longer have access to our coveted make-up counters and grooming aids - will be of utmost important to a lot of us. Not to mention a huge morale boaster.

When discussing preparedness, whether it's on my survival and preparedness for women website SurvivorJane.com, on social media networks like Facebook, Twitter, Pinterest or LinkedIn, or addressing a group or a conference, I invariably get approach by men (no, not in *that* way), and asked how they can motivate the women in their lives to get involved in disaster preparedness. What I share with these men, or anyone else for that matter, is that women are just as uncomfortable at the thought of wearing camouflage-fatigues as men would be at wearing high-heeled shoes. Which is to say, men and women speak a different language. We interpret information differently. So it could be that the approach men are using when discussing disaster preparedness has more to do with what they are talking about - guns and ammo, camouflage clothes, underground bunkers and many even a little doom and gloom. Women prefer to think about things like family, fashion, make-up and lots of good smelling things. But even if the resistance isn't the man's approach, the reluctance may simply be they don't want to give up their "woman-ness". Women love conveniences; like having their hair and nails done, and the girlie-goodies that go with them. We also like variety, like wearing different outfits each day and fixing our hair in different styles. Some of us even have a pair of shoes for every season or occasion - and in every color (guilty!) So is it really that difficult to see why some women would be reluctant to jump on the disaster preparedness wagon? To some it would mean giving up these comforts and luxuries.

୧୧୧୧୧୧୧୧୧୧୧୧୧୧୧୧୧୧୧୧୧୧୧୧୧୧୧୧୧

Self-admittingly, I was that girl. I did not want to give up the shoes, the clothes, the shopping mall trips – but more importantly ... the lifestyle. I wanted it all and I wanted it to stay just the way it was – the good with bad. It was "my" comfortable. Being oblivious to what was going on around me allowed me to stay in my 'false-sense-of-security' world. Had I taken the time to look around, there were plenty of signs that things were not as rosy as what I thought.

It wasn't until my vehicle; with me in it, were nearly car-jacked at gun-point by two people who had just robbed someone at an ATM machine, the value of my home plummeted to a fraction of its worth and, my 401k dwindled down to next to nothing that I begin to open my eyes for the first time to what was going on around me. What I saw I didn't like. This was a much darker world.

Decisions had to be made. My world as I knew it was coming to an end and I knew I may have to give up some of the conveniences I held near and dear. That was where I was stuck. I did not want to give up the heels for work-boots, my expensive hair styling accessories for a ponytail and, my manicured nails for ... well short nails and work gloves. And it seems I'm not alone. A lot of women feel this way. But I also didn't want to be forces to give these conveniences up either.

Ultimately, after a lot of thought and planning, I took a huge "leap-of-faith" and move away from the world I knew (the city) to a more rural - okay, a lot more rural, self-reliant lifestyle – for which I knew nothing about. This meant no more weekly trips to the shopping mall; no more eating out every night, and no more cleaning services for my home or clothes. I walked away from a corporate job, nice home and car and relocated to the top of a mountain, literally. This from a girl who didn't know the first thing about rural life. It was a sink or swim time.

How was I going to survive this new world and still retain my girlie-ness? Defiantly, or maybe it was pure stubbornness (okay, … it was vanity), I just couldn't throw in the towel and give up on all the "girlie goods". I began to search the internet to find ways to replace my lotions, soaps, perfumes, shampoos and conditioners. What I found surprised me – but in a good way. Most, if not all, of the products I had purchased throughout the years (and not inexpensively mind you) were originally made with things I had in my pantry and garden - really. Ingredients we been using for centuries, like oils from plant products we have or could grow in our own garden or yard; such as bay leaf, gardenia, geranium, jasmine, lavender, rose, and sage, to name a few (see nothing weird.) And moisturizers from castor oil, beeswax, sesame oil, coconut oil and olive oil; again just naming a few and again, nothing weird.

When I realized that the high-priced designer perfume I had worn for years was simply made up of 78% to 95% of specially denatured ethyl alcohol (whatever the heck that is) and essential oils, it kind of took the glamour out of it for me real quick (not to mention the thought of all that money spent!)

Armed with knowledge, I began to make my own face washes, moisturizers, and soon moved on to shampoo and conditioner. I was like a mad-scientist - experimenting with this and dabbling with that - only I wasn't mad I was actually happy! I'm not talking about mixing up chemicals, I was using items I had at the ready. And the results were amazing. Most, if not all, worked better than store bought items. I now had choices - lots of them! When I found a "good-one" I wrote it down in my "this-is-a-keeper" beauty notebook. Then, one day it dawned on me that maybe by sharing what I have learned and the fact that I haven't had to give up on the girlie things, I could help other women who were reluctant about disaster preparedness because they too were stuck on giving up these things.

ଔଔଔଔଔଔଔଔଔଔଔଔଔଔଔଔଔଔଔଔଔଔଔଔଔଔଔଔଔ

I decided to share the beauty and personal care secrets I learned by scouring the internet for skin, hair, body, and nails. Now, along with our survival food and preparedness items that will help us live as normal a life as possible should the proverbial 'poo' ever hit the fan, we also have beauty options so we don't have to resort back to looking like a cavewoman. Armed with the knowledge and ingredients found in this book we can look gorgeous any time. Just sayin'.

– Survivor Jane

CR

CONTENTS

രു

MESSAGE IN A BOTTLE ...
A MASON JAR OR GARDEN

There are items that you should consider including in your preparedness pantry and garden that will also be beneficial to your health and beauty. Although this is not an exhaustive list of items or their uses, let this serve as a guide.

Almonds - Rich source of Vitamin E, Vitamin B1, Vitamin B2, Vitamin B6, and Vitamin D. High proteins and minerals such as magnesium and calcium. High content of fats and are rich in antioxidants.

Uses: Ground almonds can be used for body scrubs and facial scrubs.

Almond Oil - Oil extract from Almonds

Uses: Used to prevents dark circles, softens skin and reduce wrinkles. Strengthens dull, damaged hair and creates shine and luster. Controls and reduces hair loss and promotes hair growth. Can be used as a carrier oil.

Aloe Vera - Belongs to garlic and onion family. Contains vitamins, minerals, amino acids, enzymes, polysaccharide, and fatty acids.

Uses: Has excellent hydrating, softening and soothing properties. Can be used as a nail strengthener. Heals and regenerates skin. Helps clear up acne and psoriasis. Acts as antimicrobials against bacteria, viruses, fungi and yeast. Good for all skin types.

Apple - Rich in alpha-hydroxy fruit acids and natural pectin.

Uses: Used in facial washes, moisturizers and facial masks.

1

ෲෲෲෲෲෲෲෲෲෲෲෲෲෲෲෲෲෲෲෲෲෲෲෲ

Apple Cider Vinegar - Contains Vitamins A, B and C, beta carotene, bioflavonoid, calcium, magnesium, potassium, phosphorus, copper, iron, sulfur, iron, fluorine, silicon, boron and pectin. Rich in antioxidants.

Uses: Used in cleansers to remove dirt and oil from skin and hair. Helps clear acne. Improves skin tone and blood circulation. Is a natural anti-aging ingredient, anti-fungal and antiseptic. Good for oily and dry complexions.

Apple Juice - Juice that has been filtered by removing apple solids.

Uses: Used for treating skin related issues like inflammation, itching, cracked skin and wrinkles.

Aspirin - Contains acetylsalicylic acid (a close relative of salicylic acid which dermatologists use to treat acne).

Uses: Used topically to reduce inflammation and remove oil and dead skin cells.

Baking Soda - Sodium bicarbonate is a natural earth mineral.

Uses: Used as an antifungal, antiseptic, exfoliant, and a deodorant.

Banana - Contains vitamins A, B, C and E and minerals potassium, zinc, iron and manganese.

Uses: Used to hydrates skin and to draw out excess fluid eliminating puffiness under eyes.

Basil - Contains antioxidant, anti-bacterial, anti-viral, adaptogenic and immune enhancing properties

CR

Uses: Used as a skin rejuvenator. Prevents appearance of blackheads. Improves skin tone. Helps maintain healthy skin and shiny hair.

Beeswax - Beeswax is a natural emulsifier. It helps reduces inflammation and soothes, hydrates, and softens skin. Has antioxidant properties.

Uses: Used in lip balms, lip glosses, hand creams, eye shadow, moisturizers, blush, eye liner, and hair pomades.

Blackberries - High in gallic acid, rutin and ellagic acid; a known chemopreventative, with anti-viral and anti-bacterial properties. High in Vitamin C.

Uses: Used in facial masks and lip balm coloring

Bran - Contains phytic acid, a B-complex vitamin and antioxidants. Rich in oil.

Uses; Used in facial cleansers, as a toners to tightens and regenerates skin. It is an effective exfoliant. Helps improve blood circulation. Stimulate cell turnover. Good for pigment balancing.

Brown Sugar - Contains calcium, magnesium, potassium and iron.

Uses: Used in facial scrubs and body scrubs as an exfoliate.

Chamomile - Contains acidic, essential oils, flavonoids and high content of Vitamin E. Has antibacterial, antifungal.

Uses: Has skin-healing properties. Soothes, softens and moisturizes skin. Has antiseptic, anti-inflammatory and anti-allergic capabilities. Helps condition and brighten hair.

CR

Canola Oil - Has naturally high levels of sterols. High in Vitamin E.

Uses: Helps skin to retain moisture.

Carrier Oils - A vegetable based oil pressed from the fatty portions of seeds, nuts or kernels. It does not evaporate. Used to dilute essential oils and absolutes before they are applied to the skin. Can be used in its pure form.

Uses: Used in pomades, conditioners, shampoos and perfumes.

Castile Soap - A mild vegetable oil-based soap saponified (made into soap) with an alkaline salt made from combination of organic extra virgin coconut, olive, jojoba and hemp oils along with pure essential oils. Completely biodegradable.

Uses: Used to make body washes, shampoos, and shaving creams.

Cinnamon - Made from the inner bark of a tropical evergreen tree, it is highly aromatic, warm and spicy. Has anti-fungal and anti-bacterial properties.

Uses: Used as a coloring agent in natural makeup powders.

Coconut Oil - Rich in fatty acids Has anti-microbial, anti-fungal and anti-protozoal properties. Helps prevent bacterial and fungal infections. Works for all skin types and hair.
Uses: Used as a natural moisturizer, to soften and protect dry, chapped skin. To treat skin irritations. It helps erase wrinkles on neck, around eyes and mouth. Rejuvenates skin.

Coffee Grounds - Contains Magnesium and Vitamin E. Acts as an antibacterial, exfoliating and stimulating agent.

CR

Uses: Used in facial scrubs and body scrubs.

Cornmeal - Obtained from ground corn. It is nutrient rich. High in niacin, minerals and linoleic acid.

Uses: Used as mild exfoliant in cosmetic formulations. It has a soothing and softening effect on the skin.

Cornstarch - Extracted starch from milled corn that is processed and dried to an ultra-fine powder.

Uses: Used in cosmetics as a natural and more healthy alternative to talc.

Cucumber - Rich in antioxidant and anti-inflammatory properties. Contains Vitamin C, beta-carotene, and manganese. An excellent protector and skin nutrient.

Uses: Used in face creams, lotions and cleansers for its astringent, soothing and cooling properties.

Cucumber Juice - Has antioxidant and anti-inflammatory properties; including vitamin C, beta-carotene, and manganese.

Uses: Used in face creams, lotions and cleansers for its astringent, soothing and cooling properties.

Egg White - Egg proteins from egg whites significantly contribute in maintaining the elasticity of skin. They are high in collagen and vitamin A.

Uses: Used in facial masks and peels.

Epsom Salt - Pure mineral compound of magnesium and sulfate. It is readily absorbed through the skin. Reduces inflammation.

છા

Uses: Used in baths and soaks and, facial treatments.

Essential Oils - Distilled from plant material. The aromatic vapor is then condensed into liquid form.

Uses: Helps revitalize skin, encouraging radiance and resilience. Used in facial washes, moisturizers, masks and peels.

Fennel Seed Oil - Oil of crushed Fennel seeds. Increases the elasticity of the connective tissues of the skin. It is anti-wrinkle and anti-aging and has a tightening effect on the skin.

Uses: Used in facial cleansers and facial masks

Garlic - Contains high levels of allicin (a sulfur). Helps cure acne scars and reduces inflammation.

Uses: Dandruff remedies, nail fungus, acnes treatments.

Glycerin - Derived from vegetable oils. Used for its ability to absorb moisture from the air. It is a humectant attracting moisture to your skin.

Uses: Used in creams, lotions and other products as a natural humectant and emollient.

Grapefruit Seed Extract - High in antioxidants, flavanoids, beta-carotene and vitamins D, C, E. and essential fatty acids such as palmitic, stearic and linoleic acid

Uses: Helps reduce wrinkles and scarring on the skin and prevent and repair skin damage. It is great for those with sensitive skin. Can help with eczema or psoriasis.

Green Tea - Powerful antioxidant inhibits the formation of cancer-causing free radicals. Helps prevent skin cell damage caused by sun exposure. Anti-inflammatory, astringent, antibacterial and anti-irritant. Slows the development of some signs of aging. Reactivates drying skin cells to improve skin condition.

Uses: Used in creams, lotions, shampoos and conditioners to soothe and moisturize skin and hair. Boosts skin's elasticity. Lightens skin. Reduces appearance of puffiness, wrinkles, fine lines and large pores.

Honey - Anti-bacterial, anti-microbial, antioxidant, and humectant. Keeps skin naturally hydrated and protected. Helps treat wounds and prevent scarring. Encourages the growth of new tissue. Makes skin soft and supple, and hair glossy and healthy. Can help treat minor acne by attacking the bacteria that cause the outbreaks while moisturizing the skin to aid rejuvenation.

Uses: Used as a thickening agent to give body to facial masks, creams, lotions, sunscreens and cleansers. Excellent skin conditioner for damaged or dry skin. Gently cleanses, soothes, softens and heals skin.

Hydrogen Peroxide - is a combination of hydrogen and oxygen. It is often used as an antiseptic to cleanse cuts, abrasions and other minor injuries (in small amounts).

Uses – Used to make natural toothpaste, as a nail soak, in hair dyes and bleaching hair treatments, and to disinfect wounds. Added to antibacterial creams and lotions, anti-aging treatments and facial products

Jojoba Oil - Has advanced molecular stability with antioxidant and anti-inflammatory actions. It is an emollient and moisturizing humectant. Helps prevent and reduce

ಣಣಣಣಣಣಣಣಣಣಣಣಣಣಣಣಣಣಣಣಣಣಣಣಣಣಣಣ

wrinkles, promotes new cell growth and makes skin luminous. Conditions hair and scalp, leaves hair shiny and lustrous. It is easily absorbed and balances sebum production.

Uses: Used in moisturizers, lotions and creams for dry skin, hair and nails. Gentle on sensitive skin. Dissolves clogged pores. Returns skin to natural pH balance. Reduces wrinkles. Helps heal scars. Beneficial to all skin types. Effective moisturizer for skin and hair.

Kiwi - Rich in omega-3 alpha- linolenic acid, vitamin C and antioxidants. Optimizes skin moisture.

Uses: Used in moisturizers, lotions and creams.

Lavender - Essential oil obtained from lavender flowers. Has antiseptic, antibacterial, antifungal and anti-inflammatory properties. Has cleansing and astringent properties. Promotes rapid healing. Slows hair loss. Has potent cell regeneration and repair capabilities.

Uses: Added to skin and hair care creams, lotions and washes for its soothing and antiseptic properties and pleasant fragrance.

Lemon - High in citric acid and Vitamin C. Has astringent, antibacterial, and antiseptic properties. Restores skins natural acid balance. Has toning properties. Exfoliates and removes oil.

Uses: Facial toners and cleaners.

Lemon Oil – Extracted from the peel of ripe lemons. Used as an stringent, antibacterial, antiseptic and cleanser. Apply to oily skin to reduce sebum production.

CR

Uses: Use to cleanse skin. Reduce wrinkles. Improve acne. Heal dry, rough, chapped skin.

Lime - High in acidity. Removes oil from the skin to fight acne. Exfoliates and helps to even out skin tone. Used as brightening agent.

Uses: Used in facial toners and exfoliants.

Mint - Anti-inflammatory, antiseptic and astringent properties. Detoxifies and clarifies skin. Natural antiseptic and freshener.

Uses: Used in facial creams, lotions, astringents and exfoliants.

Milk (powdered) - A natural cleanser high in proteins. Contains natural lactic acid. Used as mild exfoliant. Helps reduce wrinkles and improve the skin's texture. Very softening and moisturizing.

Uses: Facial exfoliants, moistures and cleansers.

Oatmeal - Contains beta glucan. High in Vitamins B and E. Rich in bran protein, potassium, phosphates, silicia, magnesium, iron. Has anti-irritant, anti-inflammatory and anti-itch properties Soothes, softens, deep cleanses, and exfoliates.

Uses: Used in exfoliants, cleaners, toners, scrubs and facial masks. Good for sensitive skin and as a cleanser for hair.

Olive Oil - High in oleic acid. Contains antioxidants, Vitamin E and polyphenols. Helps repair cells and neutralize free radicals. Has softening and smoothing properties. Helps skin hold in moisture.

CR

Uses: Facial moisturizers, creams, lotions and toners.

Onions - Helps heal acne scars. Protects against hair fall or loss. Promotes hair growth and possible re-growth.

Uses: Used in acnes treatments and hair treatments.

Orange - Good source of vitamin C. Has antiseptic properties and natural alpha-hydroxy acids (AHA). It is acidic, aromatic, uplifting, reviving and stimulating.

Uses: Facial cleansers, lotions and creams.

Orange Peel - The outer skin of the fruit. Higher Vitamin C content than the fruit. Contains Vitamin A, calcium and iron. Has aromatic, uplifting, reviving and purifying benefits.

Uses: Facial cleansers, lotions and creams

Papaya - Rich source of antioxidant nutrients such as carotenes, Vitamin C and flavonoids; B Vitamins of folate and pantothenic acid; and minerals, potassium and magnesium. Has an alpha hydroxy acid (AHA) that naturally exfoliates the skin.

Uses: Facial masks and natural exfoliant.

Peach - Rich moisturizing emollient ingredient. Contains Alpha Hydroxy Acids (AHA). Regenerate skin cell renewal. Brightens and hydrates skin.

Uses: Used in facial cleaners, toners. Unclogs pores, banishes blemishes, lighten age spots, reduces wrinkles.

Petroleum Jelly - It helps to hold in moisture and maintain existing hydration under the skin. NOTE: While petroleum jelly may be safe in its pure form, in some brands purity remains a problem, and the impurities often found in petroleum jelly, such as poly aromatic hydrocarbons (PAH), have been linked to cancer however, Vaseline brand is highly-refined, triple-purified and regarded as non-carcinogenic.

Uses: Used as a natural moisturizer to soften, and smooth lips. Moisturize eyelids. Soften hands and feet and cuticles.

Potato - Contain Vitamin C and B-Complex and minerals such as potassium, magnesium, calcium, phosphorus and zinc. Also, essential fatty acids and an assortment of phytochemicals like carotenoids and polyphenols. It is an anti-aging treatment by stimulating collagen and elastin. A skin lightener and brightener and an anti-inflammatory.

Uses: Facial masks, lotions, eye conditioners, and skin brighteners.

Pineapple - High in anti-oxidants, Vitamin C, manganese, and thiamine (Vitamin B1) and anti-inflammatory properties. The alpha hydroxyl acids give skin anti-ageing benefits.

Uses: Used in facial cleaners, lotions and exfoliants.

Pumpkin - Contains natural antioxidants, Vitamin E, and polyunsaturated fatty acids. Helps protect the skin's natural barrier and hydrates skin.

Uses: Facial masks, moisturizers and cleaners.

Rose Water A byproduct of the distillation of fresh rose petals. It is a natural hydrator and anti-irritant. Has excellent soothing agent for dry and sensitive skin.

Uses: Facial moisturizers, cleaners and lotions.

CR

Rosemary - Contains anti-oxidant, cleansing, anti-bacterial, anti-fungal, moisturizing, softening, rejuvenating properties. It is excellent for all skin types, particularly oily, acne-prone skin and eczema.

Uses: Facial cleanser and toner. Hair and scalp cleanser. Acne and blemish treatment. Hair conditioner and stimulant for hair growth.

Sage - Contains antioxidant and anti-inflammatory properties.

Uses: Used as a facial astringents and cleansers.

Sea Salt - Mineral-rich salt naturally obtained from sea water. High mineral content. An antibacterial. Exfoliates dry skin cells and opens clogged pores. Softens skin and acts as a detoxifying cleanser to draw impurities out of the body through the skin.

Uses: Used in bath soaks and body scrubs and exfoliants.

Soap nuts – Fruit produced by the sapindus plant containing large amounts of saponin (natural surfactants). Also known as soapberries.

Uses: Used as a sudsing agent for soaps.

Soapwort – Like soap nuts, contains natural saponins. Also known as Bouncing Bet

Uses: Used as a sudsing agent for soaps

Strawberries - Packed with Vitamin C, folate and sulfur. Has natural enzymes that rids the skin of impurities. Promotes new cell growth.

ෲෲෲෲෲෲෲෲෲෲෲෲෲෲෲෲෲෲෲෲෲෲෲෲ

Uses: Facial masks, lotions.

Sweet Almond Oil - Contains Vitamins A, B1, B2, B6, E, minerals, protein and is rich in essential fatty acids. Has an anti-inflammatory effect. An excellent emollient and moisturizer helps strengthens and nourishes the skin. Helps relieve itching, soreness, dryness and inflammation. Reduces reducing dark circles and puffy eyes.

Uses: Used in facial and body creams, lotions and massage oils. Beneficial for all skin types.

Tomato Juice - Contains minerals, vitamins, antioxidants and acids. Helps cleanse skin from oils, dirt, heavy makeup and dead skin cells. Has the ability to shrink pores and give skin a soft clear appearance.

Uses: Used in facial cleansers and creams.

Tea Tree Oil - An antiseptic, anti-fungal, anti-viral antimicrobial and antibacterial. Good for most skin conditions, including acne.

Uses: Used in cosmetics, dandruff shampoos, in facial masks, as moisturizer and in hair treatments.

Vegetable Oil - Good for dandruff and scalp irritation, and some kinds of hair loss. Soothing on skin.

Uses: Used for hair and skin lotions, creams and cleansers.

Vitamin E - The most potent antioxidant vitamin around. Protects skin from cancer-causing free radicals. Acts as a natural preservative in cosmetics, creams and lotions.

Uses: Used in lotions, creams, cleaners for face, body and hair.

13

ୠୠୠୠୠୠୠୠୠୠୠୠୠୠୠୠୠୠୠୠୠୠୠୠୠ

Witch Hazel - Contains cleansing, soothing, and healing properties. It is an astringent, anti-irritant, anti-inflammatory and antibacterial properties. Good for oily and troubled skin. A soothing and mild astringent that helps shrink pores.

Uses: Used in facial cleansers, toners and lotions.

Yogurt - Antibacterial and anti-fungal. Good for naturally restoring PH. High in riboflavin, calcium, protein, Vitamin B12 and lactic acid.

Uses: Facial emollient, skin conditioner, gentle cleanser and mild exfoliants.

Vodka – 100 proof Alcohol (or 80 proof) Astringent and Antibacterial. Tightens facial pores. Remove adhesive such as from band aids. Antiseptic mouthwash. Treatment for dry scalp and dandruff. Disinfectant. Mixes with essential oils.

Uses: Used as a facial astringent, Shampoos, mouthwashes and perfume. As a hand sanitizer.

❧ 1 ❧
FACIAL CARE

Women want things that are unrealistic to achieve, and we tend to go overboard trying to get there. The focus should be enhancing our natural beauty, not fighting it. - Nick Arrojo

ଔଔଔଔଔଔଔଔଔଔଔଔଔଔଔଔଔଔଔଔଔଔଔଔଔଔଔ

INVEST IN OIL

I was thinking about a post poo-hits-the-fan alternative to when I couldn't just go out and go buy my favorite face wash. What's a girl going to use to wash her delicate facial skin when there is no more facial cleaners around?' Lye soap? Uh, nooooo.

The answer? Olive Oil. I know, I know! It does sound a little counter-intuitive to put oil on your already oily face. Let alone the thought of washing with oil to remove oil? Me, like a lot of people, thought that blemishes (those awful beasts that appear on your face outta nowhere) were caused by oil. So my thinking was ..."Why on earth would anyone want to put more oil on your face?" Right?'

News Flash!! Oil is actually good for your skin! After my due diligent research, I found that soaps actually strip the oil out of your skin leaving it to repair itself by replacing the oil that we just stripped away. By washing with olive oil it replenishes the facial oil leaving you with clear skin free of blackheads, pimples, zits, whiteheads... or whatever your pet name is for those 'beasts'.

Washing your face with olive oil is nothing. In fact, Mediterranean women have used olive oil for centuries on their skin; and hair for that matter. My guess is this has something to do with the term "olive skin".

Oil actually dissolves oil. Or if you were to ask one of your nerdy chemistry friends you sat next to in school, they'd probably say "like dissolves like." You can tell I was paying attention in chemistry class. Not!

There are actually several oils that can be used and even mixed together depending on your facial skin needs. For instance, castor oil; a thicker oil, makes a great base coupled with say, olive oil or even sun flower seed oil. Experiment a little for your skin type (dry, oily, mixed et cetera).

16

ത്രെ ത്രെ ത്രെ ത്രെ ത്രെ ത്രെ ത്രെ ത്രെ ത്രെ ത്രെ ത്രെ ത്രെ ത്രെ ത്രെ ത്രെ ത്രെ ത്രെ ത്രെ ത്രെ ത്രെ

Here is the 'technique' to washing with oil. First, pour a little oil in your hand (over the sink!). Take your finger tips and apply the oil to your face, massaging it in as you go to work it deep into your pours. Next, run your wash cloth under hot steamy water (steamy not scalding mind you) and place the wash cloth over your face allowing it to cool (you know - like they do at those fancy-shmancy spas.) Once the cloth is cool, wipe the olive oil off your face. Rinse the wash cloth in hot water, and once again hold it to your face until it cools (do this a couple of times if need be.) NOTE: whatever you do, don't scrub your face – wipe it. After your little "me time" if your skin feels a little tight you can always add a drop or two of the oil and pat it on your face to absorb it.

The reason olive oil is so good for your skin is because it contains antioxidants; including flavonoids and catechins, which are also found in red wine, chocolate and, tea (all the other goodies that we love!) It also helps slow the aging process - which I am all about! In fact, I must confess, when I first started researching olive oil and its benefits, I was tempted to go out and buy the stuff by the 55 gallon drums! Just sayin'. Of course, then reality set in and I realized when the "poo" does hit the fan I would be stuck trying to move those barrels, so instead I've opted for the large box-store sizes!

As a bonus, like I mentioned before, olive oil is also great for hair and the rest of your body and can also be used as effective shaving oil too. So in one glorious bottle we can look fabulous even in a not so fabulous world!!!

FACIAL CLEANERS

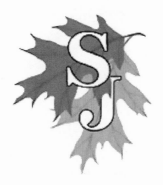

ൠൠൠൠൠൠൠൠൠൠൠൠൠൠൠൠൠൠൠൠൠൠൠൠൠ

There are four (4) different skin types with two (2) subtypes:

Normal – Skin shows neither oil nor flaking skin.

Dry – Skin feels taut or show flakes of dead skin.

Oily – Skin notably oily forehead, nose and chin – has a shiny appearance.

Combination (oily and dry) – Skin is usually oily at forehead, nose and chin and normal to dry on remainder of face.

Sensitive – Skin reacts easily to regular skin products causing redness, itchiness or a rash.

Acne-Prone – Skin is oily with the appearance of pimples (black and white heads)

ↂↂↂↂↂↂↂↂↂↂↂↂↂↂↂↂↂↂↂↂↂↂↂↂↂↂↂↂↂↂↂↂↂↂ

Milk & Honey

1 teaspoon Dark Organic Honey
1 tablespoon Whole Milk (or cream)
1 cup Water
Cotton Ball

Simmer water lightly in saucepan. Place honey in a glass mug/jar and sit it down in simmered water. When honey has melted add milk. Apply mixture to face with a cotton ball. Leave on for few minutes. Rinse.

NOTE: This is the classic milk & honey cleanser.

ↂↂↂↂↂↂↂↂↂↂↂↂↂↂↂↂↂↂↂↂↂↂↂↂↂↂↂↂↂↂↂↂↂↂ

> **Tip: milk cleans and soothes your skin**

ↂↂↂↂↂↂↂↂↂↂↂↂↂↂↂↂↂↂↂↂↂↂↂↂↂↂↂↂↂↂↂↂↂↂ

Tomato, Milk, Lemon & Orange

1 Tomato
2 tablespoons Milk
1 tablespoon Lemon Juice
1 tablespoon Orange Juice

Mix all the ingredients together. Apply to face with a cotton ball. Rinse.

ↂↂↂↂↂↂↂↂↂↂↂↂↂↂↂↂↂↂↂↂↂↂↂↂↂↂↂↂↂↂↂↂↂↂ

CR

> ## How to Wash Your Face
>
> Starting at your forehead and work your way to your nose, then outwards to your cheeks and eventually to your chin and

CRCRCRCRCRCRCRCRCRCRCRCRCRCRCRCRCRCRCRCRCRCRCRCR

Cream, Milk & Chamomile

4 tablespoons Cream
4 tablespoons Milk
 2 tablespoons Crushed Dried Chamomile Flowers
1 cup Water

Lightly simmer water in saucepan. Mix all ingredients together in a glass mug/jar and sit it down in simmered water. Let simmer for 30 minutes (don't boil). Remove from heat. Let cool for 3 hours. Strain to remove dried flowers. Apply to face. Rinse.

CRCRCRCRCRCRCRCRCRCRCRCRCRCRCRCRCRCRCRCRCRCRCRCR

Apple, Yogurt, Lime & Almond Oil

1 slice peeled Apple
2 tablespoons Plain Unflavored Yogurt (with active cultures)
1 teaspoon Almond Oil
1 teaspoon Lime Juice.

Mash apple slice. Add yogurt, almond oil and lime juice to make a paste. Apply to face. Rinse.

ℭℛℭℛℭℛℭℛℭℛℭℛℭℛℭℛℭℛℭℛℭℛℭℛℭℛℭℛℭℛℭℛℭℛ

NOTE: The apple, yogurt, lime and almond oil is natural cleanser that stimulates and revitalizes dull looking skin and, is useful for all skin types.

ℭℛℭℛℭℛℭℛℭℛℭℛℭℛℭℛℭℛℭℛℭℛℭℛℭℛℭℛℭℛℭℛℭℛ

Grapes, Milk & Olive Oil

2 tablespoons Extra Virgin Olive Oil
5 fresh Grapes
1 teaspoon Milk

Mix all ingredients into a smooth paste. Apply to face. Rinse.

NOTE: Grapes, milk and olive oil cleanses and moisturizes your skin.

ℭℛℭℛℭℛℭℛℭℛℭℛℭℛℭℛℭℛℭℛℭℛℭℛℭℛℭℛℭℛℭℛℭℛ

> **Tip: honey cleans your skin but also acts as a natural humectant which means it attracts moisture and keeps the moisture under your skin**

ℭℛℭℛℭℛℭℛℭℛℭℛℭℛℭℛℭℛℭℛℭℛℭℛℭℛℭℛℭℛℭℛℭℛ

Buttermilk & Fennel Seeds

½ cup Buttermilk
2 tablespoons Fennel Seeds (crushed)
1 cup Water

22

Simmer water lightly in saucepan. Add buttermilk and seeds in a glass jar/mug and put it down in simmered water. Let simmer 30 minutes. Remove from heat. Let cool 3 hours. Strain the seeds. Apply to face. Rinse.

NOTE: - Buttermilk and Fennel Seeds is a great cleanser for oily skin.

Tip: facial cleansers are only to cleanse the surface of your face.

Oatmeal, Honey, Cream, Lavender & Juniper Berry Oil

3 tablespoons Oatmeal Flour
1 tablespoon Dark Organic Honey
2 tablespoons Cream
2 drops Lavender Oil
2 drops Juniper Berry Oil
2 cups Water

Bring water to a light simmer in saucepan. Place cream in a glass mug/jar and put it down in simmered water. Slowly warm cream. Remove from heat. Add honey and then oatmeal. Let sit 5 minutes. Add the oils and blend. Apply to damp face. Rinse with warm water.

CR

Almonds, Cream & Lime Juice

2 tablespoons Finely Ground Almonds
1 tablespoon Cream
1 teaspoon Lime juice

Mix all ingredients together. Gently apply it to your face. Massage into skin. Rinse.

CRCRCRCRCRCRCRCRCRCRCRCRCRCRCRCRCRCRCRCRCRCR

> **Tip: low humidity (below 30%) can cause the skin on your lips, face, hands, and feet to dry and crack.**

CRCRCRCRCRCRCRCRCRCRCRCRCRCRCRCRCRCRCRCRCRCR

Corn flour, Tomato & Glycerin

2 tablespoons Corn Flour
1 tablespoon Tomato Juice
2 tablespoons Glycerin
½ glass Mineral Water
1 cup Water

Simmer water lightly in saucepan. Mix all ingredients in a glass jar/mug and put it down in simmered water. Heat mixture. Remove from heat and let cool. Apply to face. Leave on for few minutes. Rinse.

CRCRCRCRCRCRCRCRCRCRCRCRCRCRCRCRCRCRCRCRCRCR

CR

PH Balance – Scale 0-14

7 is neutral
1 - 6.9 is acidic
7.1 - 14 is alkaline
4 to 6.5 optimal

CRCRCRCRCRCRCRCRCRCRCRCRCRCRCRCRCRCRCRCRCRCRCRCR

Papaya, Aloe Vera, Honey & Yogurt

2 tablespoons Aloe Vera Gel
1 slice peeled Fresh Papaya
½ tablespoon Dark Organic Honey
1 teaspoon Plain Unflavored Yogurt (with active cultures)

Mix all ingredients together until smooth. Apply to Face. Rinse.

NOTE: Aloe Vera helps heal your skin.

CRCRCRCRCRCRCRCRCRCRCRCRCRCRCRCRCRCRCRCRCRCRCRCR

Tip: as we get older, our ability to make more natural protective oils (sebum) declines.

CRCRCRCRCRCRCRCRCRCRCRCRCRCRCRCRCRCRCRCRCRCRCRCR

CRICRICRICRICRICRICRICRICRICRICRICRICRICRICRICRICRICR

Green Tea, Cornmeal, Yogurt & Mint

1 teaspoon Green Tea
2 tablespoons Cornmeal
1 tablespoon Plain Unflavored Yogurt (with active cultures)
1 teaspoon Finely Chopped Fresh Mint leaves

Mix green tea and mint leaves. Let steep for strong tea. Cool 15 minutes. Mix tea and yogurt. Add cornmeal and let soak for a few minutes, then mix it well. Apply to face. Rinse.

CRICRICRICRICRICRICRICRICRICRICRICRICRICRICRICRICRICR

> **Tip: tomatoes are especially effective for those of us with oily skin**

CRICRICRICRICRICRICRICRICRICRICRICRICRICRICRICRICRICR

Cucumber, Oatmeal & Yogurt

½ peeled Cucumber
2 tablespoons Oatmeal
2 tablespoons Plain Unflavored Yogurt (with active cultures)

Chop and liquefy cucumber. Add remaining ingredients to cucumber liquid. Let mixture sit for a few minutes. Apply to face. Rinse.

NOTE: Cucumber, oatmeal and yogurt is a good dry skin cleanser.

CRICRICRICRICRICRICRICRICRICRICRICRICRICRICRICRICRICR

Kiwi, Yogurt, Milk, Honey, Orange, Almonds, Apricot & Lemon oil

1 peeled Kiwi Fruit
2 tablespoons Plain Unflavored Yogurt (with active cultures)
2 teaspoons Skim Milk
2 teaspoons Honey
2 teaspoons Orange Juice
1 teaspoon Finely Ground Almonds
1 teaspoon Apricot Oil
3 drops Lemon Oil (or any other citrus oil).

Peel Kiwi and mash to liquefy. Add ingredients (except the oils) to kiwi liquid. Make a paste. Slowly add oils. Apply to face. Rinse.

NOTE: Kiwi is good for dry and oily skin.

ACNE REMEDIES

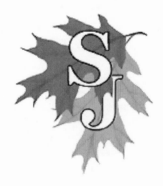

Types of Blemishes (Pimples)

Whiteheads - remain under the skin and are very small.

Blackheads - are black and appear on the surface of the skin. A blackhead is not caused by dirt.

Papules - visible on the surface of the skin. They are small bumps, usually pink.

Pustules - clearly visible on the surface of the skin. They are red at their base and have pus at the top.

Nobules - clearly visible on the surface of the skin. They are large, solid pimples. They are painful and are embedded deep in the skin.

Cysts - clearly visible on the surface of the skin. They are painful, and are filled with pus.

෴෴෴෴෴෴෴෴෴෴෴෴෴෴෴෴෴෴෴෴෴෴෴෴

Garlic

1 Garlic Clove

Mash a clove of garlic into a paste. Apply the paste directly on to the blemish. Leave on for 20 minutes. Repeat this process several times throughout the day.

NOTE: If you have dry or sensitive skin, add a few drops of milk to the garlic paste to prevent skin burning or redness.

෴෴෴෴෴෴෴෴෴෴෴෴෴෴෴෴෴෴෴෴෴෴෴෴

> Garlic is considered by some to be the holy-grail of home remedy ingredients - due in part to its powerful antioxidant, antiseptic, and antifungal properties.

෴෴෴෴෴෴෴෴෴෴෴෴෴෴෴෴෴෴෴෴෴෴෴෴

Tomato

1 Tomato

Mash a tomato into a pulp. Apply it to the blemish area and leave on for an hour. Rinse thoroughly with warm water.

෴෴෴෴෴෴෴෴෴෴෴෴෴෴෴෴෴෴෴෴෴෴෴෴

**Tip: tomatoes help
open pores**

Cucumber

¼ Cucumber

Blend cucumber into a paste. Apply directly to the blemish. Leave on for 30 minutes. Rinse off.

**Tip: consuming garlic at least
a couple times a day is also an
excellent preventive measure
against acne**

Green Tea Ice Cubes

Green Tea Ice Cubes
Wash Cloth

Pour fresh cooled green tea into ice cube trays. Freeze. Once frozen, wrap a green tea ice cube in a cloth and apply a few times throughout the day to the blemish.

ఴఴఴఴఴఴఴఴఴఴఴఴఴఴఴఴఴఴఴఴఴఴఴఴఴఴఴఴఴ

NOTE: Applying ice to inflamed blemishes not only reduces swelling and redness, but it also helps remove oil and dirt and shrink pore size.

ఴఴఴఴఴఴఴఴఴఴఴఴఴఴఴఴఴఴఴఴఴఴఴఴఴఴఴఴఴ

Tip: green tea's astringent properties promote further removal of dirt and oil.

ఴఴఴఴఴఴఴఴఴఴఴఴఴఴఴఴఴఴఴఴఴఴఴఴఴఴఴఴఴ

Baking Soda

1 tablespoon Baking Soda
Few drops Water

Mix baking soda and few drops of water to make a paste. Gently apply to the blemish and lightly scrub for a minute. Rinse with cool water.

NOTE: Baking soda gently exfoliates dead skin cells and helps loosen blackheads.

ఴఴఴఴఴఴఴఴఴఴఴఴఴఴఴఴఴఴఴఴఴఴఴఴఴఴఴఴఴ

❋ ❋ ❋

Skin Pores

Human skin has pores (tiny holes) which connect to oil glands located under the skin.

The glands are connected to the pores via follicles - small canals.

These glands produce sebum, an oily liquid.

The sebum carries dead skin cells through the follicles to the surface of the skin.

A small hair grows through the follicle out of the skin.

Blemishes grow when these follicles get blocked, resulting in an accumulation of oil under the skin.

Jojoba Oil and Tea Tree Oil

10 drops Jojoba Oil
3 drops Tea Tree Oil

Mix jojoba oil and tea tree oil together. Apply directly to blemish with cotton ball.

ℭℜ

Apple Cider Vinegar

1 teaspoon Apple Cider Vinegar
Cotton Ball

Apply apple cider vinegar to a cotton ball and apply to blemish.

ℭℜ

> **Dead skin cells, dirt, and bacteria can clog pores and cause acne**

ℭℜ

Oatmeal and Onion

3 tablespoons Plain Oatmeal
1 Medium Onion
1 oz Water

Boil water. Pour over oatmeal and let sit for five minutes. Peel onion and grind into paste. Add oatmeal. Apply to face.

ℭℜ

Mint

Fresh Mint Leaves
1 teaspoon Lemon Juice

Grind mint leaves and add lemon juice. Apply to blemish. Leave on for 15 minutes. Rinse.

NOTE: Mint acts as an astringent, clearing away pimple-causing oil.

ෞෞෞෞෞෞෞෞෞෞෞෞෞෞෞෞෞෞෞෞෞෞෞ

FACE SCRUBS
&
EXFOLIATES

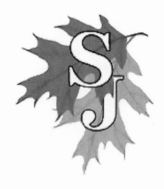

How often to use Exfoliates

Gentle Scrubs (such as sugar and plant fiber) – Safe to use every day

Coarse Scrubs (such as sea salt) – Use once a week

Oily Skin - Exfoliate two to three days a week

Dry or Sensitive Skin - Exfoliate one to two times a week with a gentle scrub.

Epsom Salt and Petroleum Jelly

2 cups Epsom Salt
1 cup Petroleum Jelly
Essential Oil (optional)

Mix Epsom Salt and Petroleum Jelly together. Add a few drops of essential oil. Apply mixture to face and gently scrub. Rinse.

જી

> ## Skin exfoliants remove dead skin cells to brighten skin

જી

Baking Soda

4 teaspoons Baking Soda
1 tablespoon Water

Mix baking soda and water to make a paste. Let sit for few minutes. Moisten face. Apply paste a gentle circular motions. Rinse.

NOTE: Baking soda gently exfoliates your skin.

જી

Tomato & Sugar

1 Tomato
½ teaspoon Brown Sugar

Cut the tomato into four sections. Dip one piece of tomato in brown sugar and gently rub it on your face. Leave on 5 minutes. Take another piece of tomato (without sugar) rub all over your face. Let it dry. Rinse.

જી

Almond, Honey & Lemon

1 tablespoon Honey
2 tablespoons Finely Ground Almonds
½ teaspoon Lemon juice.
1 cup Water

Heat water to light simmer in saucepan. Put honey in glass jar/mug and heat in water. Once honey has liquefied add ground almonds and lemon juice. Apply to face in a circular motion. Leave on 5 minutes. Rinse.

> Tip: honey cleans your skin but also acts as a natural humectant.

Sea Salt, Olive Oil and Honey

2 tablespoons Sea Salt
1 tablespoon Extra-Virgin Olive Oil
1 tablespoon Honey

Mix ingredients together. Apply to face in circular motion. Rinse

NOTE: Honey will attract water and seal it into the skin.

Aspirin

5-7 uncoated Aspirin
Water

Crush the aspirin into powder. A water to make a paste. Apply to face in circular motion. Leave on 10 minutes. Rinse.

છા

NOTE: The salicylic acid in the aspirin removes dead skin cells while conditioning the skin.

છા

> **Tip: if you exfoliate too much you can damage your skin.**

છા

Honey, Almonds, Oatmeal, and Lemon Juice (or Yogurt)

1 tablespoon Honey
1 tablespoon Finely Ground Almonds
2 tablespoons Dry Oatmeal
Few drops of Lemon Juice (or Yogurt)

Combine honey, ground almonds, oatmeal and lemon juice. Make a paste. Massage on face. Rinse.

છા

Brown Sugar, Olive Oil, Oats, Cinnamon and Nutmeg

½ cup Brown Sugar
2 tablespoons Extra Virgin Olive Oil
2 teaspoons Instant Oats
½ teaspoon Ground Cinnamon
½ teaspoon Ground Nutmeg

CR

Mix brown sugar, olive oil, oats, cinnamon and nutmeg to make a paste. Apply to face. Leave on 2 minutes. Rinse.

Oatmeal, Powdered Milk,
and Cornmeal

1 cup of Ground Oatmeal
2 teaspoon Cornmeal
½ cup of Powdered Milk

Mix oatmeal, powdered milk and cornmeal in bowl. Place in container with lid. To use combine mix 1 tablespoon of mixture with enough water to make paste. Apply to face. Massage in circular motions. Rinse.

CRCRCRCRCRCRCRCRCRCRCRCRCRCRCRCRCRCRCRCRCRCRCR

Tip: sea salt exfoliates, detoxifies and cleanses

CRCRCRCRCRCRCRCRCRCRCRCRCRCRCRCRCRCRCRCRCRCRCR

Papaya and Pineapple

1 Papaya
½ Pineapple

Cube papaya and pineapple. Mash and press cubes through a sieve to extract juice. Using a cotton ball apply juice to face. Leave on for 15 minutes. Rinse.

CRCRCRCRCRCRCRCRCRCRCRCRCRCRCRCRCRCRCRCRCRCRCR

41

⊗⊗⊗⊗⊗⊗⊗⊗⊗⊗⊗⊗⊗⊗⊗⊗⊗⊗⊗⊗⊗⊗⊗⊗⊗⊗⊗⊗⊗

Brown Sugar and Olive Oil

½ cup of Brown Sugar
3 tablespoons of Olive Oil
Water

Mix brown sugar, olive oil and a few drops of water into a paste. Apply to face in circular motion. Rinse.

⊗⊗⊗⊗⊗⊗⊗⊗⊗⊗⊗⊗⊗⊗⊗⊗⊗⊗⊗⊗⊗⊗⊗⊗⊗⊗⊗⊗⊗

> **Tip: oatmeal and baking soda sloughs off dead skin cells making your skin glow**

⊗⊗⊗⊗⊗⊗⊗⊗⊗⊗⊗⊗⊗⊗⊗⊗⊗⊗⊗⊗⊗⊗⊗⊗⊗⊗⊗⊗⊗

Oatmeal and Baking Soda

2 tablespoons Oatmeal
1 teaspoon Baking Soda
Water

Combine oatmeal, baking soda and enough water to make a paste. Gently apply to face in a circular motion. Rinse with warm water.

⊗⊗⊗⊗⊗⊗⊗⊗⊗⊗⊗⊗⊗⊗⊗⊗⊗⊗⊗⊗⊗⊗⊗⊗⊗⊗⊗⊗⊗

భిళి

MOSITURIZERS

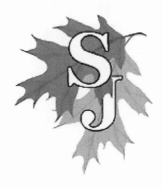

Moisturizers for Skin Types

Normal Skin: Light, Non-greasy Moisturizers

Dry Skin: Heavy, Oil-based Moisturizers

Oily Skin: Light, Water-based Moisturizers

Sensitive Skin: Soothing Non-irritant Moisturizers

Mature Skin: Oil-based Moisturizers

Strawberries and Lemon Juice

Strawberries
1 tablespoon Lemon Juice
½ cup Cream

Mash strawberries. Add lemon juice and cream to make paste. Apply to face. Leave on 20 minutes. Rinse.

Oatmeal, Aloe Vera and Honey

¼ cup Cooked Oatmeal
1 tablespoon Aloe Vera Gel
2 tablespoons Honey

CR

Mix the ingredients together to make a paste. Apply to face. Gently rub in circular motion. Rinse.

CRCRCRCRCRCRCRCRCRCRCRCRCRCRCRCRCRCRCRCRCRCRCRCR

Whole Milk, Egg Yolk and Grape Seed

1 Egg Yolk
¼ cup Whole Milk
1 tablespoon Grape Seed Oil.

Mix the ingredients together to make a cream. Apply to face. Rinse.

CRCRCRCRCRCRCRCRCRCRCRCRCRCRCRCRCRCRCRCRCRCRCRCR

Apple and Honey

Apple
½ tablespoon Honey

Peel, core and mash apple. Mix honey to apple and make a paste. Apply to face. Rinse.

NOTE: Apple and honey is a nourishing face pack for oily skin.

CRCRCRCRCRCRCRCRCRCRCRCRCRCRCRCRCRCRCRCRCRCRCRCR

Tip: the best way to apply moisturizer is on damp skin. Wash your face and pat it - then apply the moisturizer on the face and lips.

Yogurt, Honey Lemon and Egg White

½ a Lemon
1 ½ teaspoon Honey
3 tablespoons Yogurt
1 Egg White

Squeeze the juice from lemon. Add honey and yogurt. Whip the egg white and add to mixture. Apply to face. Leave on 15 minutes. Rinse.

Coconut Oil, Honey, and Lemon Juice

Coconut Oil
Honey
Lemon Juice

Mix coconut oil, honey and lemon juice in equal parts. Apply to face. Rinse.

Ground Almonds and Olive Oil

2 tablespoons Ground Almonds
2 tablespoons Olive Oil

Combine ground almonds with olive oil. Apply to your face in a gentle circular motion. Rinse well.

Avocado/Almond Oil, Beeswax and Vitamin E

1 cup Almond or Avocado Oil
½ cup Beeswax
3 capsules of Vitamin E
Essential Oils (optional)

In a saucepan heat almond oil and beeswax on low heat. Once wax melts remove from heat and stir. Let cool. Add Vitamins E and a few drops of essential oil. Apply to face. Rinse.

> **Moisturizers hold water in the outermost layer of skin**

Peach, Coconut, Almond oil, Orange Oil and Rose Water

Peach
1 tablespoon Coconut Oil
1 teaspoon Almond Oil
¼ teaspoon Orange Oil
¼ teaspoon Rose Water

Peel, pit and mash peach into a pulp. Strain through a sieve. Add oils, peach juice and rose water together. Apply to face. Rinse.

C3CR

Olive Oil, Coconut Oil, Vegetable Oil, Vitamin E and Strawberries

1 tablespoon Olive Oil
1 tablespoon Coconut Oil
1 tablespoon Vegetable Oil
2 drops of Vitamin E Oil
2 tablespoon Strawberries (mashed)

Mix mashed strawberries and oils together. Apply to face. Rinse.

CRCRCRCRCRCRCRCRCRCRCRCRCRCRCRCRCRCRCRCRCRCRCRCR

> If you have sensitive skin be cautious of ingredients that call for fruits that contain citric acids.

CRCRCRCRCRCRCRCRCRCRCRCRCRCRCRCRCRCRCRCRCRCRCRCR

Olive Oil, Lemon Juice and Egg

2 tablespoons of Olive Oil
½ a teaspoon of Lemon Juice
Egg

Mix olive oil, lemon juice and beaten egg. Apply to face. Rinse.

NOTE: This Olive Oil moisturizer is best suited for dry skin.

CRCRCRCRCRCRCRCRCRCRCRCRCRCRCRCRCRCRCRCRCRCRCRCR

CR

Tip: choose the best moisturizer for your face by skin type, age and skin conditions (such as acne or sensitivity)

CRCRCRCRCRCRCRCRCRCRCRCRCRCRCRCRCRCRCRCRCRCRCR

Lime Juice, Milk & Olive Oil

Lime Juice
¼ cup Milk
2 tablespoons Olive Oil

Boil milk. Add juice squeezed from juice and then olive oil. Cool slightly. Apply to face. Rinse.

CRCRCRCRCRCRCRCRCRCRCRCRCRCRCRCRCRCRCRCRCRCRCR

Sweet Almond Oil

Small amount Sweet Almond Oil
3 drops of Water (distilled)

Mix sweet almond with water. Apply to face. Rinse.

NOTE: Apply sweet almond oil to face regularly to keep it moist.

CRCRCRCRCRCRCRCRCRCRCRCRCRCRCRCRCRCRCRCRCRCRCR

CR

Lemon Juice, Egg White, Honey and Strawberry

1 tablespoon Lemon Juice
2 tablespoons Egg White
2 tablespoons Honey
½ cup Mashed Strawberries

Mix all ingredients together. Into a paste. Apply to face. Rinse.

CRCRCRCRCRCRCRCRCRCRCRCRCRCRCRCRCRCRCRCRCRCRCRCR

Dehydrated Apricots and Milk Powder

Dehydrated Apricots
2 tablespoons Skimmed Milk Powder

Rehydrate apricots until soft. Blend apricots with skimmed milk powder. Apply to face. Leave on 15 minutes. Rinse.

CRCRCRCRCRCRCRCRCRCRCRCRCRCRCRCRCRCRCRCRCRCRCRCR

> **Oatmeal has fantastic skin treating properties**

CRCRCRCRCRCRCRCRCRCRCRCRCRCRCRCRCRCRCRCRCRCRCRCR

Oatmeal and Honey

2 tablespoons Cooked Oatmeal
1 teaspoon Honey

Mix cooked oatmeal with honey. Apply to face. Rinse.

CR

NOTE: Honey can be used as a minor acne treatment as well.

CRCRCRCRCRCRCRCRCRCRCRCRCRCRCRCRCRCRCRCRCRCRCRCRCR

Yogurt, Orange Juice and Lemon Juice

1 cup Yogurt
1 teaspoon Orange Juice
1 teaspoon Lemon Juice

Mix yogurt, lemon juice and orange juice. Apply to face. Rinse.

CRCRCRCRCRCRCRCRCRCRCRCRCRCRCRCRCRCRCRCRCRCRCRCRCR

Banana

½ Banana (ripe)

Mash banana until creamy. Apply to face. Leave on 20 minutes. Rinse.

CRCRCRCRCRCRCRCRCRCRCRCRCRCRCRCRCRCRCRCRCRCRCRCRCR

Honey

1 tablespoon Honey

Apply honey to face. Leave on 10 minutes. Rinse.

CRCRCRCRCRCRCRCRCRCRCRCRCRCRCRCRCRCRCRCRCRCRCRCRCR

Yogurt and Honey

1 tablespoon Yogurt
1 tablespoon Honey

51

Mix yogurt and honey. Apply to moist face. Leave on 15 minutes. Rinse.

NOTE: Yogurt and honey moisturizes, hydrates and soothes the skin.

Olive Oil, Lemon Juice and Egg White

1 tablespoon Olive Oil
1 tablespoon Lemon Juice
1 Egg White

Mix olive oil, lemon juice and egg white. Apply to face. Leave on 15 minutes. Rinse.

Honey, Oatmeal and Aloe Vera Gel

2 tablespoon Honey
¼ cup Oatmeal (cooked)
1 tablespoon Aloe Vera Gel

Mix honey, oatmeal and aloe vera gel. Apply to face. Rinse.

Apple and Honey

Apple
½ tablespoon Honey

Peel, deseed and mash apple. Add honey and make a paste. Apply to face. Rinse.

NOTE: Apple and Honey are good for oily skin.

> ## Your skin is a barrier against many bacterial and viral infections

Honey, Lemon, Yogurt and Egg White

1 ½ teaspoon Honey
½ teaspoon Lemon
3 tablespoons Yogurt
Egg White (whipped)

Mix honey, lemon and yogurt. Mix in egg white. Apply to face. Leave on 15 minutes. Rinse.

Vegetable Oil, Honey and Lemon Juice

1 teaspoon Vegetable Oil
1 teaspoon Honey
½ teaspoon Lemon Juice

Combine vegetable oil, honey and lemon juice into a paste. Apply to face. Leave on 10 minutes. Rinse.

FACIAL MASKS

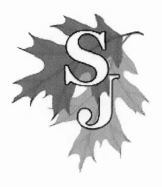

Banana, Lemon and Honey

1 Banana (small)
1 teaspoon Honey
8 drops of Lemon Juice

Mash banana. Add honey and lemon juice and mix well. Apply to face. Leave on 10 minutes. Rinse.

Dried Chamomile Flowers, Bran and Honey

1 tablespoon Dried Chamomile Flowers
¾ cup Water
2 tablespoon Bran
1 teaspoon Honey (warmed)

Boil water. Pour water over the chamomile flowers. Steep 30 minutes. Strain to remove dried flowers. Warm honey and mix 3 tablespoons of liquid. Add bran and mix well. Apply to face. Leave on 15 minutes. Rinse.

Strawberries and Egg Yolk

¼ cup Strawberries
1 Egg Yolk (beaten)

Mash strawberry and add beaten egg yolk. Apply to face. Leave on 10 minutes. Rinse.

CR

Honey and Milk

2 tablespoons Honey
2 teaspoons Milk

Mix honey and milk into a paste. Apply to face. Leave on for 20 minutes. Rinse.

CRCRCRCRCRCRCRCRCRCRCRCRCRCRCRCRCRCRCRCRCRCR

Pumpkin, Yogurt, Honey, Almonds and Olive Oil

2 cups Pumpkin (pureed, cooked fresh or canned)
4 tablespoons Unflavored Yogurt
4 tablespoons Honey
1/3 cup ground Almonds
¼ teaspoons Olive Oil

Mix pumpkin, yogurt, honey, ground almonds, and olive oil. Apply to face. Leave on 10 minutes. Rinse.

CRCRCRCRCRCRCRCRCRCRCRCRCRCRCRCRCRCRCRCRCRCR

> Pumpkins are rich in Vitamins A and C along with various enzymes that help nourish and brighten skin.

CRCRCRCRCRCRCRCRCRCRCRCRCRCRCRCRCRCRCRCRCRCR

CR

Oatmeal Egg and Honey

1 tablespoon Honey
1 Egg Yolk
Oatmeal

Mix honey and egg yolk. Add oatmeal to create a thick paste.
Apply to face. Leave it on 15 minutes. Rinse.

CRCRCRCRCRCRCRCRCRCRCRCRCRCRCRCRCRCRCRCRCRCRCRCR

Blackberry and Sour Cream

2-3 Blackberries
2 tablespoons Sour Cream

Mash blackberries. Add sour cream and make a paste. Apply to face.
Leave on 10 minutes. Rinse.

CRCRCRCRCRCRCRCRCRCRCRCRCRCRCRCRCRCRCRCRCRCRCRCR

Peach, Honey and Yogurt

1 Large Peach
3 teaspoon Honey
2 tablespoons Yogurt

Peel, pit and mash the peach. Mix peach and honey together. Add
yogurt and make a paste. Apply to face. Leave on for 10 minutes.
Rinse.

CRCRCRCRCRCRCRCRCRCRCRCRCRCRCRCRCRCRCRCRCRCRCRCR

Raspberry, Oatmeal, Olive Oil
and Grape Seed Oil

1 teaspoon Olive Oil
1 teaspoon Grape Seed Oil

꙰꙰꙰꙰꙰꙰꙰꙰꙰꙰꙰꙰꙰꙰꙰꙰꙰꙰꙰꙰꙰꙰꙰꙰꙰꙰꙰꙰꙰꙰

2 tablespoons Oatmeal Powder (ground oatmeal)
2-3 Raspberries

Mix olive oil, grape seed oil, oatmeal powder and raspberries. Make a paste. Apply to face. Leave on 20 minutes. Rinse.

꙰꙰꙰꙰꙰꙰꙰꙰꙰꙰꙰꙰꙰꙰꙰꙰꙰꙰꙰꙰꙰꙰꙰꙰꙰꙰꙰꙰꙰꙰

Note: The antioxidant rich pack of raspberries, olive oil and grape seed oil, helps in getting rid of wrinkles, freckles and fine-lines.

꙰꙰꙰꙰꙰꙰꙰꙰꙰꙰꙰꙰꙰꙰꙰꙰꙰꙰꙰꙰꙰꙰꙰꙰꙰꙰꙰꙰꙰꙰

Chamomile Tea and Oatmeal

½ cup Fresh Chamomile Tea
¼ cup Oatmeal

Mix chamomile tea and oatmeal. Let sit 2-3 minutes. Apply to face. Leave on 20 minutes. Rinse.

꙰꙰꙰꙰꙰꙰꙰꙰꙰꙰꙰꙰꙰꙰꙰꙰꙰꙰꙰꙰꙰꙰꙰꙰꙰꙰꙰꙰꙰꙰

FACIAL PEELS

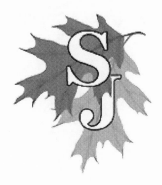

꙾꙾꙾꙾꙾꙾꙾꙾꙾꙾꙾꙾꙾꙾꙾꙾꙾꙾꙾꙾꙾꙾꙾꙾꙾꙾꙾꙾

Alpha Hydroxyl Acids (AHA) and **Beta Hydroxyl Acids** (BHA) are mild chemical exfoliants extracted from things like citrus fruits, sugar cane and willow bark.

AHAs and BHAs work by buffing away dead surface cells to uncover the healthier skin beneath.

Alpha Hydroxyl Acids (AHA):
Water-Soluble
Used to treat Dry Skin

Beta Hydroxy Acids (BHA):
Lipid-Soluble
Used for Oily Complexions

꙾꙾꙾꙾꙾꙾꙾꙾꙾꙾꙾꙾꙾꙾꙾꙾꙾꙾꙾꙾꙾꙾꙾꙾꙾꙾꙾꙾

Gelatin, Milk, Essential Oil, and Tea Tree Oil

1 tablespoon of Gelatin (Powdered or Granulated)
1-2 tablespoons of Milk
Few drops of Essential Oil (optional)
1 cup Water

Mix gelatin and milk in an glass bowl/jar. Heat water to a light simmer. Sit glass jar/mug down into hot water until gelatin is melted. Add essential oil.. Apply to face with tongue depressor. Leave on 30 minutes. Peel mask off.

CR

> **Tip: use tongue depressor, popsicle stick or small spatula to apply ingredients.**

CRCRCRCRCRCRCRCRCRCRCRCRCRCRCRCRCRCRCRCRCRCRCRCRCR

Gelatin, Lemon and Orange

1 Packet Gelatin (unflavored)
Juice of 1 Lemon
Juice of 1 Orange

Heat lemon juice and orange juice together in saucepan. Add gelatin. Let cool slightly. Apply to face. Peel mask off when dry.

NOTE: As the gelatin dries it firms and tones.

CRCRCRCRCRCRCRCRCRCRCRCRCRCRCRCRCRCRCRCRCRCRCRCRCR

> **Aspirin is a source of salicylic acid, a type of BHA**

CRCRCRCRCRCRCRCRCRCRCRCRCRCRCRCRCRCRCRCRCRCRCRCRCR

Gentle Fruit Peel

1 cup Pineapple
½ cup Papaya
1 tablespoon Honey

ଔଔଔଔଔଔଔଔଔଔଔଔଔଔଔଔଔଔଔଔଔଔଔଔଔଔଔଔ

Mash pineapple and papaya together. Add honey and make a paste. Apply to face. Peel mask off when dry.

ଔଔଔଔଔଔଔଔଔଔଔଔଔଔଔଔଔଔଔଔଔଔଔଔଔଔଔଔ

Cucumber, Egg White and Lemon Juice

¼ Cucumber (peeled and seeded)
1 Egg White
1 teaspoon Lemon Juice

Mash cucumber. Add egg white and lemon juice with cucumber to make a paste. Apply to face. Peel mask off when dry.

ଔଔଔଔଔଔଔଔଔଔଔଔଔଔଔଔଔଔଔଔଔଔଔଔଔଔଔଔ

> **Cucumber diminishes hyperpigmentation, and reduces fine lines and wrinkles**

ଔଔଔଔଔଔଔଔଔଔଔଔଔଔଔଔଔଔଔଔଔଔଔଔଔଔଔଔ

Tomato, Gelatin, and Orange Juice

1 Tomato (pulp only)
1 package Gelatin (unflavored)
1 tablespoon Orange Juice

Wash face. Heat orange juice, tomato pulp and gelatin. Mix into a paste. Let cool slightly. Apply to face. Peel mask off when dry.

NOTE: Tomatoes helps to restore the natural PH of the skin.

ଔଔଔଔଔଔଔଔଔଔଔଔଔଔଔଔଔଔଔଔଔଔଔଔଔଔଔଔ

CR

Tip: facial peels exfoliate dead skin cells, reduce blackheads, soften your skin, even out the tone and reduce wrinkling

CRCRCRCRCRCRCRCRCRCRCRCRCRCRCRCRCRCRCRCRCRCRCRCR

Egg, Honey, Citrus Juice, and Gelatin

1 Egg (yolk)
1 teaspoon Honey
1/8 cup Citrus Juice (Lemon, Orange or Lime)
1 Packet Gelatin (unflavored)

Wash face. Mix ingredients together into a paste. Apply to face. Peel mask off when dry.

CRCRCRCRCRCRCRCRCRCRCRCRCRCRCRCRCRCRCRCRCRCRCRCR

Avocado, Honey and Egg

¼ of an Avocado
1 teaspoon Honey
1 Egg White- (beaten)

Whip egg white until stiff. Add honey and avocado. Make a paste. Apply to face. Peel mask off when dry.

CRCRCRCRCRCRCRCRCRCRCRCRCRCRCRCRCRCRCRCRCRCRCRCR

FACIAL TONERS

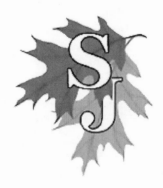

CR

Aloe Vera and Thyme

1 cup Aloe Vera Juice
2 teaspoons Thyme

Combine aloe vera juice with thyme. Let it set over night. Strain out thyme keeping the liquid. Apply liquid to face with a cotton ball.

CRCRCRCRCRCRCRCRCRCRCRCRCRCRCRCRCRCRCRCRCRCRCRCRCR

> **Tip: you will get the most out of your facial toner if you wash your face first**

CRCRCRCRCRCRCRCRCRCRCRCRCRCRCRCRCRCRCRCRCRCRCRCRCR

Basil

¼ cup fresh Basil
1 cup Water

Soak fresh basil in boiling water for 15 minutes. Let cool. Strain liquid and pour into spray type bottle. Apply to face using a cotton ball.

CRCRCRCRCRCRCRCRCRCRCRCRCRCRCRCRCRCRCRCRCRCRCRCRCR

Olive Oil and Alpha Lipoic Acid

1 teaspoon Olive Oil
250 mg Alpha Lipoic Acid
(cont'd)

ෆෆෆෆෆෆෆෆෆෆෆෆෆෆෆෆෆෆෆෆෆෆෆෆෆ

Heat olive oil. Empty a capsule of alpha lipoic acid and mix together. Massage it into your face. Leave on 5 minutes.

ෆෆෆෆෆෆෆෆෆෆෆෆෆෆෆෆෆෆෆෆෆෆෆෆෆ

Apple Cider Vinegar and Aspirin

½ oz Apple Cider Vinegar
5 Aspirins (uncoated)
4 oz Water

Mix apple cider vinegar and water. Finely crush aspirins. Add aspirins to vinegar mixture. Use a cotton ball and wipe on face.

ෆෆෆෆෆෆෆෆෆෆෆෆෆෆෆෆෆෆෆෆෆෆෆෆෆ

Toners – are made of water and are skin soothers. Aloe or chamomile plant oils, cleanse and draw moisture to the skin.

Fresheners – most are alcohol-free.

Astringents - usually for oily skin and designed to fight acne or control oil.

ෆෆෆෆෆෆෆෆෆෆෆෆෆෆෆෆෆෆෆෆෆෆෆෆෆ

Apple and Witch Hazel

1 Apple (peeled)
½ cup Water

66

CR

¼ cup Witch Hazel

Peel, deseed and cube apple. Place in saucepan with water. Bring to boil and remove from the heat. Let mixture cool completely. Strain out the apple. Add witch hazel. Apply to face with cotton ball.

CRCRCRCRCRCRCRCRCRCRCRCRCRCRCRCRCRCRCRCRCRCRCRCR

Different Toners for Skin Types

Some help remove excess dirt and oil from your face.

Some soothe skin and help to restore the skin's pH balance.

Some condition your skin.

CRCRCRCRCRCRCRCRCRCRCRCRCRCRCRCRCRCRCRCRCRCRCRCR

Lemon Juice Witch Hazel and Rubbing Alcohol

¼ cup Lemon Juice
1/3 cup Witch Hazel
2 Tablespoons Rubbing Alcohol
½ cup Water

Mix lemon juice, witch hazel, alcohol and water. Pour into a container. Apply to face with cotton ball when needed.

CRCRCRCRCRCRCRCRCRCRCRCRCRCRCRCRCRCRCRCRCRCRCRCR

ANTI-WRINKLE

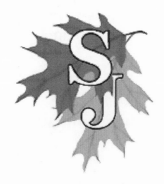

CR

Cocoa Butter, Honey, Apricot Oil
and Sesame Oil

1 tablespoon Cocoa Butter
½ tablespoon Honey
2 drops of Sesame Oil
2 drops of Apricot Oil

Mix ingredients together into a cream. Apply to face. Leave on 15 minutes. Rinse.

CRCRCRCRCRCRCRCRCRCRCRCRCRCRCRCRCRCRCRCRCRCRCRCRCRCR

Carrot, Potato, Turmeric and Baking Soda

1 small Carrot
1 small Potato
¼ teaspoon Turmeric
¼ teaspoon Baking Soda

Cut carrot and potato into small pieces and boil in saucepan. Once softened removed from heat. Mash into a paste. Add turmeric and baking soda and mix well. Apply to face. Leave on 20 minutes. Rinse.

CRCRCRCRCRCRCRCRCRCRCRCRCRCRCRCRCRCRCRCRCRCRCRCRCRCR

> Carrots are a rich source of Vitamin A, which helps in booting the collagen production of skin.

CRCRCRCRCRCRCRCRCRCRCRCRCRCRCRCRCRCRCRCRCRCRCRCRCRCR

ひらひらひらひらひらひらひらひらひらひらひらひらひらひらひらひら

Honey, Yogurt, Lemon Juice, Vitamin E and Turmeric

1 teaspoon Honey
2 teaspoons Yogurt
1 teaspoon Lemon Juice
1 capsule Vitamin E
¼ teaspoon Turmeric

Mix all ingredients into a paste. Apply to face. Leave on 15 minutes. Rinse.

ひらひらひらひらひらひらひらひらひらひらひらひらひらひらひらひら

> Lemon juice contains Vitamin C which is very effective in treating wrinkles.

ひらひらひらひらひらひらひらひらひらひらひらひらひらひらひらひら

Potato

1 Potato (small)

Grate potato. In sieve press out liquid. Using cotton ball apply the liquid to face.

ひらひらひらひらひらひらひらひらひらひらひらひらひらひらひらひら

Orange Juice, Pear, Apple, Strawberries and Grapes

1 oz Orange Juice
½ Pear
½ Apple
2-3 Strawberries

CR

2-3 Grapes
Honey

Mash apple, pear, strawberries and grapes. Add orange juice and make a paste. Apply a thin coat of honey to your face. Spread fruit mixture to face. Leave on 30 minutes. Rinse.

CRCRCRCRCRCRCRCRCRCRCRCRCRCRCRCRCRCRCRCRCRCRCRCRCRCRCR

Coconut Oil and Vitamin E

¼ teaspoon Coconut Oil
2 drops Vitamin E

Mix coconut oil and vitamin E. Apply to face and let it absorb.

CRCRCRCRCRCRCRCRCRCRCRCRCRCRCRCRCRCRCRCRCRCRCRCRCRCRCR

Wrinkling in the skin is promoted by habitual facial expressions, aging, sun damage, smoking, poor hydration, and various other factors

CRCRCRCRCRCRCRCRCRCRCRCRCRCRCRCRCRCRCRCRCRCRCRCRCRCRCR

Castor Oil and Lemon Juice

¼ teaspoon Castor Oil
Few drops Lemon Juice

Mix castor oil and lemon juice and apply to wrinkle areas.

ભૂ

> ## Pure castor oil when used regularly can help prevent wrinkles

ભૂ

Jojoba Oil, Apricot Kernel Oil, Rosehip Seed Oil, Carrot Seed Essential Oil and Beeswax

3 teaspoons Jojoba Oil
3 teaspoons Apricot Kernel Oil
3 teaspoons Rosehip Seed Oil
5 drops Carrot-Seed Essential Oil
1 ½ teaspoons Beeswax
5 teaspoons Rose-Water (optional)

Heat 1 cup of water to a light simmer in saucepan. Place beeswax, jojoba, rosehip and apricot oils in a glass jar/mug. Heat until wax is melt. Remove from heat. Add remaining ingredients and stir well. Pour into container with lid. Place in cool place. Use under eyes in the morning and evening.

ભૂ

Honey

1 teaspoon Honey

Apply honey to a cleansed face. Leave on 10 minutes. Rinse.

ભૂ

NOTE: Honey will draw out skin impurities and moisturize skin

രു

An anti-wrinkle cream is a compound
formulated to help restore moisture and
elasticity to skin and help to minimize or hide
the presence of wrinkles

രു

Olive Oil

2-3 drops Olive Oil

Apply olive oil to face. Gently rub it into skin.

NOTE: Olive Oil is good for dry skin

രു

Orange Juice

¼ teaspoon Orange Juice
Cotton Balls

Soak a cotton pad in orange juice. Apply to face. Rinse

രു

Walnuts, Yogurt and Almond Oil

2 Walnuts
2 tablespoons Yogurt
1 teaspoon Almond Oil

෯෯෯෯෯෯෯෯෯෯෯෯෯෯෯෯෯෯෯෯෯෯෯෯෯෯෯

Finely crush walnuts. Add walnuts to yogurt and almond oil. Apply to face. Rinse.

NOTE: Walnuts, yogurt and almond oil are gentle enough to use everyday

෯෯෯෯෯෯෯෯෯෯෯෯෯෯෯෯෯෯෯෯෯෯෯෯෯෯෯

Egg

Egg White

Separate the yolk. Apply egg white to face. Leave on 10 minutes. Rinse.

NOTE: Egg white is good for oily skin

෯෯෯෯෯෯෯෯෯෯෯෯෯෯෯෯෯෯෯෯෯෯෯෯෯෯෯

Black Tea

2 tablespoon Black Tea (brewed)
Wash Cloth

Saturate wash cloth with warm black tea. Lie down and place cloth over face. Leave on 10 minutes.

෯෯෯෯෯෯෯෯෯෯෯෯෯෯෯෯෯෯෯෯෯෯෯෯෯෯෯

❧ 2 ❧
EYE CARE

*Beauty is in the eye of
the beholder*

EYE PUFFINESS
DARK CIRCLES
&
UNDER EYE BAGS

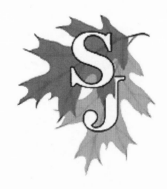

CR

Potato

1 Potato

Finely grate a potato into a bowl. Mash to make it slightly liquefied. Lie down. Gently massage potato mixture under eyes. Leave on 15 minutes.

NOTE: Potatoes have natural properties that help reduce swelling.

CRCRCRCRCRCRCRCRCRCRCRCRCRCRCRCRCRCRCRCRCRCRCRCRCR

> Puffy eyes are caused by fluid retention, genetics, allergic reaction, dehydration or hormones

CRCRCRCRCRCRCRCRCRCRCRCRCRCRCRCRCRCRCRCRCRCRCRCRCR

Silverware Spoons

2 Metal Silverware Spoons

Chill the spoons in a glass of ice water. Place a spoon on each eye.

NOTE: The cool metal of the spoons constricts the blood vessels which helps decrease redness and puffiness around the eyes.

CRCRCRCRCRCRCRCRCRCRCRCRCRCRCRCRCRCRCRCRCRCRCRCRCR

CR

Causes for Dark Circles Under the Eye

Genetics - when blood pools because of slower circulation it causes fragile capillaries to stretch and leak making it more obvious with those with thin skin under the eyes.

Age - over time skin loses collagen and thins causing the veins under the eyes to become more noticeable.

Seasonal Allergies - Allergies trigger the release of histamines in the body, which inflame blood vessels and cause swelling under the eyes.

CRCRCRCRCRCRCRCRCRCRCRCRCRCRCRCRCRCRCRCRCRCRCRCR

Green Tea

2 Green Tea Bags (Black or Green Best)

Steep two tea bags in hot water for 5-10 seconds. Place tea bags in plastic baggie. Once cool apply tea bags over your eyes for 15 minutes.

CRCRCRCRCRCRCRCRCRCRCRCRCRCRCRCRCRCRCRCRCRCRCRCR

CR

Apple Cider Vinegar and Potato

2 tablespoons Apple Cider Vinegar
Grated Potato

Mix apple cider with grated potatoes. Lie down. Pack mixture on eyes and cover with a warm cloth. Leave on 20 minutes. Rinse with warm water.

CRCRCRCRCRCRCRCRCRCRCRCRCRCRCRCRCRCRCRCRCRCRCRCRCR

Cucumber

2 Slices Cucumber

Lie down. Apply a slice of cucumber on each eye. Leave on for 15 minutes.

CRCRCRCRCRCRCRCRCRCRCRCRCRCRCRCRCRCRCRCRCRCRCRCRCR

Almond Oil and Honey

¼ teaspoon Almond Oil
¼ teaspoon Honey

Combine almond oil and honey. Apply under your eyes.

CRCRCRCRCRCRCRCRCRCRCRCRCRCRCRCRCRCRCRCRCRCRCRCRCR

Cold Compress

Ice Cubes
Wash Cloth

Wrap ice cubes in a wash cloth, or soak a wash cloth in cold water, or use a frozen bag. Place over eyes. Leave on 10 – 15 minutes.

EYE LASH CONDITIONERS

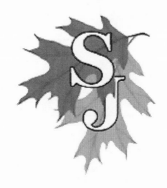

CR

Coconut Oil, Vitamin E, and Sweet Almond Oil

Coconut Oil
Vitamin E
Sweet Almond Oil

Mix small amounts of all the oils together. Apply to lashes with a clean cotton swab at night. Remove in the morning.

CRCRCRCRCRCRCRCRCRCRCRCRCRCRCRCRCRCRCRCRCRCRCR

Tip: clean and disinfect a used mascara tube and the wand and pour oil in the tube for easy application.

CRCRCRCRCRCRCRCRCRCRCRCRCRCRCRCRCRCRCRCRCRCRCR

Petroleum Jelly

Petroleum Jelly

Apply a small amount of petroleum jelly on eyelashes at night. Remove in the morning.

CRCRCRCRCRCRCRCRCRCRCRCRCRCRCRCRCRCRCRCRCRCRCR

Castor Oil and Lemon Zest

2-4 oz Castor Oil
1 tablespoon Lemon Zest

ରେ ରେ

Pour the castor oil into a small bottle with a screw on lid. Add the lemon zest and allow to sit for several days. Apply to lashes at night. Remove in morning.

ରେ ରେ

> Upper lid has about 200 lashes. The lower lid has about 100

ରେ ରେ

Green Tea

Cooled Green Tea

Apply cool green tea to your lashes with a cotton ball or swab.

ରେ ରେ

> Green tea is rich in flavonoids, including epigallocatechin-3-gallate, which has potent antioxidant and health-supportive effects

ରେ ରେ

Lemon Peel and Olive Oil

Lemon Peel
Olive Oil

CR

Pour olive oil in a small jar with lid and add lemon peel. Let sit for several days. Apply to lashes with cotton swab at night. Remove in morning.

CRCRCRCRCRCRCRCRCRCRCRCRCRCRCRCRCRCRCRCRCRCRCRCR

NOTE: Lemon is a mild natural antiseptic and antimicrobial agent, and may help promote healthier lashes.

CRCRCRCRCRCRCRCRCRCRCRCRCRCRCRCRCRCRCRCRCRCRCRCR

A human eyelash "lives" for about 90 days.

CRCRCRCRCRCRCRCRCRCRCRCRCRCRCRCRCRCRCRCRCRCRCRCR

Almond/Castor Oil and Vanilla Extract

¾ teaspoon Almond Oil (or Castor Oil)
¼ teaspoon Vanilla Extract

Mix almond oil and vanilla extract. Pour mixture into a small jar or bottle. Apply to lashes with cotton swab.

CRCRCRCRCRCRCRCRCRCRCRCRCRCRCRCRCRCRCRCRCRCRCRCR

Olive Oil and Sage

1 teaspoon Extra Virgin Olive Oil
2 cups Fresh Sage Leaves (or 1 cup of dried sage leaves)
1 cup Water

Combine sage leaves and water in a saucepan. Bring water to a boil. Simmer for 15 minutes. Remove from heat and cool. Strain liquid into a jar or bottle with lid. Add olive oil and shake well. Apply to lashes using cotton swab.

Vitamin E Oil, Olive Oil, and Vanilla Extract

¼ teaspoon Olive Oil
¾ teaspoon Vitamin E Oil
Few drops Vanilla Extract

Combine vitamin E oil and olive oil. Pour into small jar or bottle with lid. Add vanilla extract. Apply with cotton swab.

EYE SOOTHERS
&
RELAXERS

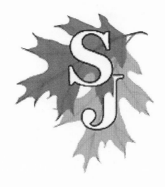

CR

Cucumber

2 Cucumber Slices

Apply one slice of cucumber to each eye. Let sit for twenty minutes, then remove.

CRCRCRCRCRCRCRCRCRCRCRCRCRCRCRCRCRCRCRCRCRCR

> **The skin around the eye area is thin and very sensitive**

CRCRCRCRCRCRCRCRCRCRCRCRCRCRCRCRCRCRCRCRCRCR

Cucumber Juice

1-2 Cucumber Slices

Extract juice from cucumber slices. Gently apply juice with cotton ball to eye area. Leave on 15 minutes. Rinse.

CRCRCRCRCRCRCRCRCRCRCRCRCRCRCRCRCRCRCRCRCRCR

Peach

1 Ripe Peach

Peel, pit and mash peach into a smooth paste. Gently apply paste under eyes. Leave on 20 minutes. Rinse.

CRCRCRCRCRCRCRCRCRCRCRCRCRCRCRCRCRCRCRCRCRCR

CR

Mint

Fresh Mint Leaves

Grind leaves and small amount of water to make paste. Apply to the eye area. Leave on 20 minutes. Rinse.

CRCRCRCRCRCRCRCRCRCRCRCRCRCRCRCRCRCRCRCRCRCRCRCRCR

> Eye soothers help diminishes the appearance of puffiness, dark circles and signs of fatigue

CRCRCRCRCRCRCRCRCRCRCRCRCRCRCRCRCRCRCRCRCRCRCRCRCR

Cucumber, Aloe Vera Gel, Cornstarch, and Witch Hazel

1 teaspoon Cucumber Juice
1 tablespoon Aloe Vera Gel
¼ teaspoon Corn Starch
Few drops Witch Hazel

Mix cucumber juice, aloe vera gel and corn starch together in small saucepan. Lightly simmer. Remove from heat. Add witch hazel and mix well. Let it cool. Place in jar/bottle. Apply to skin under the eye.

CRCRCRCRCRCRCRCRCRCRCRCRCRCRCRCRCRCRCRCRCRCRCRCRCR

Egg White and Lemon Juice

1 Egg White
3-5 Drops Lemon Juice

CR

Mix egg white with lemon juice. Saturate two clean cotton balls in the mixture. Squeeze excess liquid out. Lie down. Place over the eyes and leave on 10 minutes. Rinse.

CRCRCRCRCRCRCRCRCRCRCRCRCRCRCRCRCRCRCRCRCRCRCRCRCR

Avocado and Almond Oil

3 Ripe Avocados
5-6 Drops Almond Oil

Mash avocados. Add almond oil and make a paste. Lie down. Apply to area around the eye. Leave on 10 minutes. Rinse.

CRCRCRCRCRCRCRCRCRCRCRCRCRCRCRCRCRCRCRCRCRCRCRCRCR

Aloe Vera Gel and Cucumber

¼ Cucumber
2 oz Aloe Vera Gel

Mash cucumber. Strain through a sieve. Combine aloe vera gel and 1 tablespoon of cucumber juice. Pour into a bottle or jar and chill. Apply area around the eye.

CRCRCRCRCRCRCRCRCRCRCRCRCRCRCRCRCRCRCRCRCRCRCRCRCR

Pomegranate Seed Oil, Grape Seed Oil, Carrot Seed Oil, and Wheatgerm Oil

1 tablespoon Grape Seed Oil (cont'd)
1 teaspoon Pomegranate Seed Oil
1 teaspoon Carrot Seed Oil
1 teaspoon Wheatgerm

Combine oils. Place in a jar or bottle. Use a few drops under eyes.

❧ 3 ❧
HAND CARE

*Anyone who keeps the ability to
see beauty never grows old. ~
Franz Kafka*

HAND CREAMS
&
EXFOLIATES

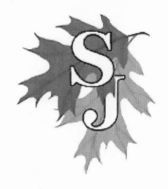

Almonds, Honey, Walnut/Sunflower Oil and Lemon Juice

1 oz Ground Almonds
1 teaspoon Honey
2 teaspoons Walnut or Sunflower Oil
1 teaspoon Lemon Juice

Mix all ingredients into a thick paste. Apply to hands. Gently rub for 2-3 minutes. Rinse.

Sugar, Apricot Oil, Lemon Juice/Lemon Essential Oil

½ cup Sugar
2 tablespoons Apricot Oil
½ a Lemon (or 3 drops lemon essential oil)

Combine sugar, apricot oil, and lemon juice. Rub mixture on hands for 2-3 minutes. Rinse.

NOTE: Apricot oil is a natural lubricant.

Tip: to keep moisture in your hands wear a pair of light cotton gloves on your hands at night after applying hand treatment

෬෬෬෬෬෬෬෬෬෬෬෬෬෬෬෬෬෬෬෬෬෬෬෬෬෬෬

Almond, Oats, Yogurt, Almond Oil
and Lemon Juice

1 teaspoon Almonds
2 teaspoons Rolled Oats
1 tablespoon Yogurt
1 teaspoon Almond Oil
1 teaspoon Lemon Juice

Grind the almonds and oats until finely ground. Add remaining ingredients. Massage onto damp hands. Leave on 15 minutes. Rinse.

෬෬෬෬෬෬෬෬෬෬෬෬෬෬෬෬෬෬෬෬෬෬෬෬෬෬෬

Coconut Oil, Shea Butter, Cocoa Butter, Aloe Vera Juice, Sweet
Almond Oil and Essential Oil

¼ cup Coconut Oil
1/8 cup Shea Butter
1/8 cup Cocoa Butter
1 tablespoon Aloe Vera Juice
1 tablespoon Sweet Almond Oil)
5-10 drops essential oils (optional)
1 cup Water

Heat water to a light simmer. In a glass jar/mug combine coconut oil, shea butter and cocoa butter. Sit glass jar into water. When melted remove from heat. Add aloe vera juice and sweet almond oil. Pour into container and let cool. Apply to hands.

෬෬෬෬෬෬෬෬෬෬෬෬෬෬෬෬෬෬෬෬෬෬෬෬෬෬෬

> One of the first places to show age
> is our hands

CR

Sweet Almond Oil, Coconut Oil, Olive Oil, Beeswax and Essential Oils

1/3 cup Sweet Almond Oil
2 tablespoons Coconut Oil
2 tablespoons Olive Oil
3 tablespoons Beeswax (grated)
30-35 drops Essential Oil

Mix oils in a small saucepan to warm. Remove from heat. Add grated beeswax and completely melt. Cool slightly. Add essential oil. Poured cream into a container and completely cool. Apply to hands.

CRCRCRCRCRCRCRCRCRCRCRCRCRCRCRCRCRCRCRCRCRCR

Safflower Oil and Sugar

2 tablespoons Safflower Oil (or Olive Oil)
3 tablespoons Sugar (coarse)

Mix safflower oil and sugar into a paste. Gently rub mixtures on hands. Rinse.

CRCRCRCRCRCRCRCRCRCRCRCRCRCRCRCRCRCRCRCRCRCR

Sea Salt, Olive Oil and Baking Soda

¾ cup Sea Salt (coarse)
¼ cup Olive Oil
1 teaspoon Baking Soda

Mix sea salt, olive oil and baking soda. Pour in tight sealed container. Gently rub on hands. Rinse.

CRCRCRCRCRCRCRCRCRCRCRCRCRCRCRCRCRCRCRCRCRCR

Brown Sugar, Almond Oil, Calendula Oil, Tea Tree Oil and Lime Juice

2 cups Brown Sugar
1 cup Almond Oil
20 drops Calendula Oil
10 drops Tea Tree Oil
2 tablespoons Lime Juice

Mix brown sugar, almond oil, calendula oil, tea tree oil and lime juice into a paste. Pour mixture into a container with lid. Gently apply exfoliant to hands. Gently rub for 2 minutes. Rinse.

BROWN SPOT REMOVER

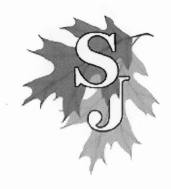

Causes for Brown Spots (also known as Liver Spots)

Sun/UV Light: the sun/UV light is the biggest cause of discolorations of the skin.

Pregnancy: due to hormonal changes

Blemishes: blemishes can cause scarring and dark spots.

Medications – certain medications can cause dark spots

Lemon Juice

Lemon Juice (or lemon slice)

Apply lemon juice directly to brown spot. Leave on 30 minutes. Rinse. Or, place lemon slice to the area for 15 minutes.

CR

Milk

Milk

Apply milk to brown spot with cotton ball.

NOTE: Lactic acid in milk can help speed cell turnover which can help fade spots quicker.

CRCRCRCRCRCRCRCRCRCRCRCRCRCRCRCRCRCRCRCRCRCRCRCRCR

Lemon Juice

½ teaspoon Sugar
1 teaspoon Lemon Juice

Combine sugar and lemon juice. Apply to brown spot. Leave on 30 minutes. Rinse.

CRCRCRCRCRCRCRCRCRCRCRCRCRCRCRCRCRCRCRCRCRCRCRCRCR

Buttermilk

4 teaspoons Buttermilk
2 teaspoons Tomato Juice

Apply buttermilk directly to brown spot. Leave on for 2-3 minutes. Rinse.

NOTE: Buttermilk contains more lactic acid than regular milk.

CRCRCRCRCRCRCRCRCRCRCRCRCRCRCRCRCRCRCRCRCRCRCRCRCR

෪෪෪෪෪෪෪෪෪෪෪෪෪෪෪෪෪෪෪෪෪෪෪෪෪෪෪෪

Yogurt

Yogurt (plain)

Apply yogurt directly on brown spot. Leave on 20 minutes. Rinse.

෪෪෪෪෪෪෪෪෪෪෪෪෪෪෪෪෪෪෪෪෪෪෪෪෪෪෪෪

Tip: remember, it took time to develop brown spots and it will take time to erase them as well

෪෪෪෪෪෪෪෪෪෪෪෪෪෪෪෪෪෪෪෪෪෪෪෪෪෪෪෪

Castor Oil

Castor Oil

Apply castor oil with a cotton ball on to the brown stop. Gently massage.

NOTE: Castor Oil has strong healing properties

෪෪෪෪෪෪෪෪෪෪෪෪෪෪෪෪෪෪෪෪෪෪෪෪෪෪෪෪

Red Currants

¼ cup Red Currants (unripen)
1 tablespoon Honey

Mashed red currants. Add honey and mix well. Apply to brown spot. Leave 30 minutes. Rinse

Aloe Vera Gel

Aloe Vera Gel

Apply aloe vera gel to brown spot. Rub gently. Leave on 30 minute. Rinse.

Apple Cider Vinegar and Onion Juice

1 tablespoon Apple Cider Vinegar
1 tablespoon Onion Juice

Finely chop onion. Strain in a sieve. Add onion liquid and apple cider vinegar. Apply to brown spot.

❧ 4 ❧
NAIL CARE

*Beautiful nails are
jewels - not tools*

NAIL STRENGTHENERS

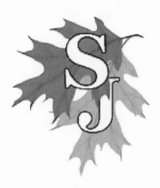

How to give yourself a manicure

Starting with clean hands and nails.

File nails to same length.

Soak nails in warm soapy water to soften cuticles.

Push cuticles back with an orange stick.

Apply a base coat to all nails to protect the nail and help the nail polish to go on smoothly.

Next apply the nail polish. Begin by polishing a thin layer down the center of the nail and then one down each side.

Wait a few minutes, then apply a second coat of polish.

Lastly, apply a clear top coat.

Let nails dry.

ରେ

Lemon Juice

Lemon Juice
Water

Mix lemon juice and water. Apply to nails with cotton ball. Leave on for a few minutes. Rinse.

ରେ

Toothpaste and Lemon Juice

Toothpaste
Lemon Juice

Mix toothpaste with a few drops of lemon juice. Scrub nails with toothpaste to remove stains and add shine.

NOTE: Lemon Juice is a natural bleaching agent.

ରେ

Petroleum Jelly

Apply petroleum jelly to nails after washing hands.

NOTE: Finger nails contain no fat and cannot naturally hold moisture.

ରେ

Honey, Egg Yolks and Milk

1 tablespoon Honey
2 Egg Yolks
¼ cup Milk

03CR03CR03CR03CR03CR03CR03CR03CR03CR03CR03CR03CR03CR03CR03CR03CR03

Combine honey, beaten egg yolks, and milk. Soak nails for 10-15 minutes. Rinse.

NOTE: Honey, egg yolks and milk contain natural proteins and calcium to help strengthen and reinforce the structure of the nail

03CR03CR03CR03CR03CR03CR03CR03CR03CR03CR03CR03CR03CR03CR03CR03CR03

Castor Oil, Salt, and Wheat Germ Oil

2 teaspoons Castor Oil
2 teaspoons Salt
1 teaspoon Wheat Germ Oil

Mix all ingredients. Pour into jar with lid. Apply to each nail. Leave on 5 minutes. Wipe with cotton ball.

03CR03CR03CR03CR03CR03CR03CR03CR03CR03CR03CR03CR03CR03CR03CR03CR03

Olive Oil and Lemon Juice

3 tablespoons Olive Oil
1 tablespoon Lemon Juice
1 cup Water

Bring water to a light simmer. In a glass jar/mug mix olive oil and lemon juice. Place jar into water to warm. Remove from heat. Apply with cotton ball.

03CR03CR03CR03CR03CR03CR03CR03CR03CR03CR03CR03CR03CR03CR03CR03CR03

Apple Cider Vinegar

4 tablespoons Apple Cider Vinegar

Pour apple cider vinegar into a bowl. Soak finger nails for 2-3 minutes . Rinse.

Salt

1 tablespoon Salt
Water (cold)

Combine salt and water in a bowl. Soak finger nails 2-3 minutes. Rinse.

NAIL
CONDITIONERS

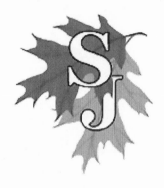

CA

Vinegar

4 tablespoons Vinegar.

Pour vinegar into bowl. Soak finger nails for 2-3 minutes. Rinse.

CACACACACACACACACACACACACACACACACACACACACACA

Listerine

4 tablespoons Listerine

Pour Listerine into bowl. Soak finger nails for 2-3 minutes. Rinse.

NOTE: Listerine is a powerful antiseptic

CACACACACACACACACACACACACACACACACACACACACACA

> ## Tip: dry or damaged nails require special treatment.

CACACACACACACACACACACACACACACACACACACACACACA

Garlic

1 Garlic Clove

Crush garlic clove to liquefy. Apply directly to nails. Leave on 2-3 minutes. Rinse.

CACACACACACACACACACACACACACACACACACACACACACA

Hydrogen Peroxide

4 tablespoons Hydrogen Peroxide (3%)

Pour Hydrogen Peroxide into bowl. Soak nails 2-3 or until nails are clean.

Salt Water

1 tablespoon Salt

Add salt to bowl of water. Soak nails 2-3 minutes. Rinse

NOTE: Soaking nails in salt water can help prevent bacteria and fungus from infiltrating the nail bed.

Vicks Vapor Rub

1/8 teaspoon Vapor Rub

Apply a thick layer of vicks vapor rub to your nail if you have developed a fungus

✺ 5 ✺
FOOT CARE

There is no foot too small that it cannot leave an imprint on this world.

FOOT CREAMS

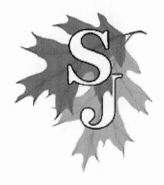

Beeswax, Cocoa Butter, Coconut Oil, Sweet Almond Oil, Lemon Essential Oil, and Ginger Essential Oil

½ oz Beeswax
½ oz Cocoa Butter
2 oz Coconut Oil
2 tablespoons Sweet Almond Oil
1 ½ teaspoon Lemon Essential Oil
½ teaspoon Ginger Essential Oil
4 tablespoons Mineral Water

Heat oils, beeswax and cocoa butter in a saucepan over low heat. Add water a little at a time. Mix well. Remove from heat. Slightly cool. Add essential oils. Let cool completely. Put in jar and store in dark place. Use on feet as needed.

Strawberries, Apricot Oil and Sea Salt

8-10 Strawberries
2 tablespoons Apricot Oil
1 teaspoon Sea Salt (coarse)

Mash strawberries. Add apricot oil and sea salt. Apply to feet and gently rub. Rinse.

FOOT
POWDERS

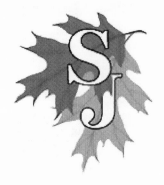

Cornstarch, Baking Soda and Peppermint Essential Oil

½ cup Cornstarch
½ cup of Baking Soda
12 to 14 drops Peppermint Essential Oil

Mix all ingredients together. Let dry 12 hours. Store in airtight container. Use as needed.

Corn Flour, Lavender Oil and Tea Tree Oil

2 tablespoons Corn Flour
15 drops Lavender Oil
5 drops Tea Tree Oil

Place corn flour in a bottle. Add lavender oil and tea tree oil. Let sit at least 24 hours. Shake well before using. Use as needed.

Cornstarch, Baking Soda, Baking Powder and Lavender Essential Oil

1 cup Cornstarch
½ cup Baking Soda
½ cup Baking Powder
Few drops Lavender Essential Oil

Mix all dry ingredients. Add essential oil. Place in container with lid. Use as needed.

NOTE: Lavender is an antibacterial.

ଔଔଔଔଔଔଔଔଔଔଔଔଔଔଔଔଔଔଔଔଔଔଔଔଔଔଔଔଔ

Baking Soda, Tea Tree Oil, Peppermint Oil and Cornstarch

5 cups Baking Soda
25 drops Tea Tree Oil
15 drops of Peppermint Oil
½ a cup of Cornstarch

Combine baking soda, tea tree oil, and peppermint oil. Mix into a fine powder. Add cornstarch and mix well. Store in container with lid. Use as needed.

ଔଔଔଔଔଔଔଔଔଔଔଔଔଔଔଔଔଔଔଔଔଔଔଔଔଔଔଔ

> **Tip: to make a real fine foot powder use a flour sifter.**

ଔଔଔଔଔଔଔଔଔଔଔଔଔଔଔଔଔଔଔଔଔଔଔଔଔଔଔଔ

Baking Soda, Borax, and Clove Essential Oil

3 tablespoons Baking Soda
1 tablespoon Borax
10 drops Clove Essential Oil (or Rosemary Essential Oil)

Combine ingredients together. Story in an airtight container.

NOTE: Clove essential oil and rosemary essential oil are both antimicrobial

ଔଔଔଔଔଔଔଔଔଔଔଔଔଔଔଔଔଔଔଔଔଔଔଔଔଔଔଔ

TOENAIL FUNGUS REMEDIES

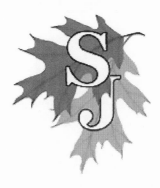

෨ଓଓଓଓଓଓଓଓଓଓଓଓଓଓଓଓଓଓଓଓଓଓଓଓଓଓ

> General hygiene practices such as
> keeping toe nails short, dry and
> clean by regular trimming will help
> decrease the risk of infection.

෨ଓଓଓଓଓଓଓଓଓଓଓଓଓଓଓଓଓଓଓଓଓଓଓଓ

Lavender Oil, Tea Tree Oil
and Apple Cider Vinegar

10 drops Lavender Oil
6 drops Tea Tree Oil
4 teaspoons Apple Cider Vinegar
1/8 cup Water

Boil water in saucepan. Mix lavender oil, tea tree oil, and apple cider
vinegar to water. Apply to affected areas with cotton 3 times daily.

෨ଓଓଓଓଓଓଓଓଓଓଓଓଓଓଓଓଓଓଓଓଓଓଓଓ

> **Tip: turmeric is a spice with
> a natural enzyme that fights nail
> fungus**

෨ଓଓଓଓଓଓଓଓଓଓଓଓଓଓଓଓଓଓଓଓଓଓଓଓ

CR CR CR CR CR CR CR CR CR CR CR CR CR CR CR CR CR CR CR CR CR CR CR

Tea Tree Oil and Apple Cider Vinegar

1 cup Apple Cider Vinegar
12 drops Tea Tree Oil
1 cup Water

Mix warm apple cider vinegar, with tea tree oil, and warm water. Soak feet 10-20 minutes several times a week to kill fungus.

CR CR CR CR CR CR CR CR CR CR CR CR CR CR CR CR CR CR CR CR CR CR CR

What is Athletes Foot?

It's a fungal infection of the foot.

Usually develops between the toes.

Requires a warm and moist environment to develop.

Contagious to other areas of the body.

Can be treated with antifungal treatments.

To avoid - keep feet clean and dry

CR CR CR CR CR CR CR CR CR CR CR CR CR CR CR CR CR CR CR CR CR CR CR

Oregano Essential Oil and Olive Oil

2 drops Oregano Essential Oil
1 teaspoon Olive Oil

117

Mix oregano oil and olive oil. Rub on afflicted area every day for 3 weeks.

 Tip: oregano essential oil is a powerful antiseptic and fungicide

Tea Tree Oil and Olive Oil

1 drops Tea Tree Oil
1 drop Olive Oil

Apply tea tree oil with olive oil directly to infected toe nails.

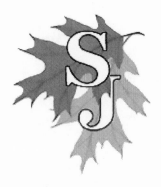

FOOT SOAKS

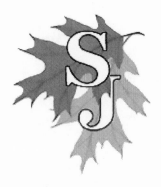

෨෨෨෨෨෨෨෨෨෨෨෨෨෨෨෨෨෨෨෨෨෨෨෨෨෨

Essential Oils for Foot Soaks

Relaxing:
Bergamot, Frankincense, Geranium, Lavender, Lime, Patchouli, Rosewood, Sandlewood, and Ylang Ylang

Refreshing:
Lemongrass, Lime, Manuka, Orange and Spearmint

Antiseptic:
Eucalyptus, Lavender, Manuka and Tea Tree

Antibacterial:
Eucalyptus Lavender, and Tea Tree

Antifungal:
Eucalyptus, Peppermint, Sandalwood And Tea Tree

෨෨෨෨෨෨෨෨෨෨෨෨෨෨෨෨෨෨෨෨෨෨෨෨෨෨

Apple Cider Vinegar

2 capfuls of Apple Cider Vinegar

Add apple cider vinegar to a warm foot bath to relieve and revive tired feet.

CR

Listerine, Vinegar and Water

¼ cup Listerine
¼ cup Vinegar
½ cup Warm Water

Mix Listerine, vinegar and warm water. Add to warm foot bath. Soak 10 minutes.

CRCRCRCRCRCRCRCRCRCRCRCRCRCRCRCRCRCRCRCRCRCRCRCR

Epsom Salt, Baking Soda and Essential Oil

1 ½ tablespoons Epsom Salt
1 ½ tablespoons Baking Soda
Few drops of Essential Oil (optional)

Add ingredients to a gallon of warm/hot water. Soak for 10 minutes.

CRCRCRCRCRCRCRCRCRCRCRCRCRCRCRCRCRCRCRCRCRCRCRCR

Chamomile Tea, Dried Parsley and Essential Oil

4 bags Chamomile Tea
1/8 cup Dried Parsley
4 drops Essential Oil

Add ingredients to one gallon of hot water. Let steep for 10 minutes before using.

CRCRCRCRCRCRCRCRCRCRCRCRCRCRCRCRCRCRCRCRCRCRCRCR

Kosher Salt, Epsom Salts and Essential Oil

2 cups Kosher Salt
1 cup Epsom Salts
Few drops Essential Oil (optional)

ରେଇତ୍ରାଇତ୍ରାଇତ୍ରାଇତ୍ରାଇତ୍ରାଇତ୍ରାଇତ୍ରାଇତ୍ରାଇତ୍ରାଇତ୍ରାଇତ୍ରାଇ

Mix ingredients together. Add 2 -3 tablespoons to a gallon of water. Soak for 10 minutes.

ରେଇତ୍ରାଇତ୍ରାଇତ୍ରାଇତ୍ରାଇତ୍ରାଇତ୍ରାଇତ୍ରାଇତ୍ରାଇତ୍ରାଇତ୍ରାଇତ୍ରାଇ

> **Tip: add marbles or smooth river rocks to the bottom of your foot soak to rub your feet over while soaking.**

ରେଇତ୍ରାଇତ୍ରାଇତ୍ରାଇତ୍ରାଇତ୍ରାଇତ୍ରାଇତ୍ରାଇତ୍ରାଇତ୍ରାଇତ୍ରାଇତ୍ରାଇ

Epsom Salts, Kosher Salt, Baking Soda, and Cornstarch

1 ¼ cups Epsom Salts
1 ¼ cups Kosher Salt
¼ cup Baking Soda
¼ cup Cornstarch

Mix ingredients together. Add 2 - 3 tablespoons to a gallon of warm /hot water. Soak for 10 minutes.

ରେଇତ୍ରାଇତ୍ରାଇତ୍ରାଇତ୍ରାଇତ୍ରାଇତ୍ରାଇତ୍ରାଇତ୍ରାଇତ୍ରାଇତ୍ରାଇତ୍ରାଇ

Lemon Juice, Olive Oil and Milk

1 cup Lemon Juice
3 tablespoons Olive Oil
¼ cup Milk

Combine ingredients. Add 2 -3 tablespoons to a gallon of warm/hot water. Soak for 10 minutes.

⊱ 6 ⊰
BODY CARE

Nothing makes a woman more beautiful than the belief she is beautiful. ~*Sophia Loren*

Common Skin Conditions

Eczema - a chronic inflammatory skin disorder which runs in families and is often associated with a history of asthma and allergies.

Contact eczema/dermatitis – caused an allergen or irritant touches the skin.

Irritant contact dermatitis – a developing rash from soaps, detergents, harsh products or prolonged contact with mild irritants like bubble bath or even sweat.

Allergic eczema/contact dermatitis - an allergic reaction in the skin from a specific substance such as poison ivy, poison sumac and poison oak, or metals such as nickel used for accessories and jewelry.

ଔଔଔଔଔଔଔଔଔଔଔଔଔଔଔଔଔଔଔଔଔଔଔଔଔଔ

SURVIVAL BATHING

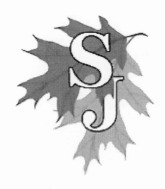

CR

Sponge Bath

Bowl
Wash Cloth
Soap
Water

Add water into a bowl. Dip washcloth into it. Put soap on washcloth and wash over your body. Rinse the soap off of the washcloth and repeat.

CRCRCRCRCRCRCRCRCRCRCRCRCRCRCRCRCRCRCRCRCRCRCR

1 Gallon Water Bath

Large Bowl (or Bucket)
Cup
Wash Cloth
Soap
Water

Fill bowl with water. Put head down in water to get wet and wash hair with soap/shampoo. Rinse hair over the bowl by dipping a cup into water and pouring it over head letting water go back into bowl. Take a sponge bath with the remaining water.

CRCRCRCRCRCRCRCRCRCRCRCRCRCRCRCRCRCRCRCRCRCRCR

Water Bottle Bath

Water Bottle
Water
Soap

Pour a small amount of water out of the bottle into your hands and wet your body, or wet a wash cloth. Lather body with soap. Pour more water in hands/wash cloth to rinse off.

NOTE: Punch a hole in the top of the water bottle cap to avoid pouring out too much water at one time.

Garden/Yard Sprayer

1 Gallon Garden Sprayer (with adjustable spray nozzle)
Water
Soap

Take a clean garden sprayer and fill to the fill-line with clean water. Spray your body down with water. Lather yourself with soap. Rinse with sprayer.

NOTE: For warm water, place the garden sprayer in a black plastic garbage bag and sit it out in the sun during the day.

BODY WASHES

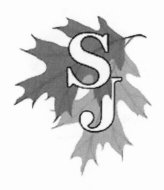

Essential Oils for Skin

Chamomile - Good for dry and sensitive skin, acne, eczema, and dermatitis.

Geranium – Good for oily complexions, acne, mature skin, eczema, and dermatitis.

Grapefruit - Extremely cleansing for oily skin.

Lavender – Good for all skin types.

Palmarosa - Stimulates new cell growth, moisturizes skin, and regulates oil production.

Patchouli - Antimicrobial, astringent, fungicidal, and deodorant. Good for acne, dry skin, eczema, and oily skin

Peppermint – Has astringent properties.

Rosemary - Useful for acne, eczema, and dermatitis.

Sandalwood – Useful for acne, dry, skin.

Sweet Orange – Good for dull or oily skin.

Tea tree – Antibacterial. Useful oil for acne, oily skin, rashes, and inflamed skin.

Ylang ylang – Great for general skin care, irritated skin, oily skin, or acne.

ඣඣඣඣඣඣඣඣඣඣඣඣඣඣඣඣඣඣඣඣඣඣඣඣඣඣඣඣ

Castile Soap, Glycerine and Essential Oil

1 cup water
¼ cup liquid castile soap
1 teaspoon vegetable glycerine
12-15 drops of essential oils (optional)

Mix all ingredients together and pour into bottle. Wet skin. Apply to wash cloth or hand and bathe. Rinse.

ඣඣඣඣඣඣඣඣඣඣඣඣඣඣඣඣඣඣඣඣඣඣඣඣඣඣඣ

Castile Soap, Honey, Grape Seed Oil, Vitamin E
And Essential Oil

⅔ cup liquid castile soap
¼ cup raw, unfiltered honey
2 teaspoons Grape Seed Oil (or jojoba oil, sweet almond oil, sesame seed oil, olive oil)
1 teaspoon Vitamin E oil
50 – 60 drops Essential Oils

Combine all ingredients. Mix well. Pour in squirt bottle. Wet skin. Apply to wash cloth or hand and bathe. Rinse.

ඣඣඣඣඣඣඣඣඣඣඣඣඣඣඣඣඣඣඣඣඣඣඣඣඣඣඣ

BODY SCRUBS

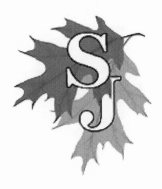

ෲෲෲෲෲෲෲෲෲෲෲෲෲෲෲෲෲෲෲෲෲ

Brown Sugar, Sea Salt, Coconut/Olive Oil, Honey, and Lemon Juice

1 cup Brown Sugar
½ cup Sea Salt
2 tablespoons Coconut Oil (or Olive Oil)
1 tablespoon Honey
2 tablespoons Lemon Juice
1 tablespoon Essential Oil

Mix brown sugar, sea salt, coconut oil , honey, lemon juice and essential oil into a paste. Apply to moist skin in circular motion. Rinse.

ෲෲෲෲෲෲෲෲෲෲෲෲෲෲෲෲෲෲෲෲෲ

> Skin is the largest organ of your body

ෲෲෲෲෲෲෲෲෲෲෲෲෲෲෲෲෲෲෲෲෲ

Fresh Coffee Grounds and Salt

3 tablespoons Fresh Coffee Grounds
1 tablespoon salt

Brew a fresh pot of coffee. Mix coffee grounds and salt. Scrub mixture over body. Rinse.

ෲෲෲෲෲෲෲෲෲෲෲෲෲෲෲෲෲෲෲෲෲ

NOTE: Coffee contains magnesium and Vitamin E and acts as an antibacterial, exfoliating and stimulating agent.

Strawberries, Honey, Wheat Bran, Yogurt and Essential Oil

½ cup Yogurt
½ cup Strawberries
1 tablespoon Honey
½ cup Wheat Bran
5 drops Lavender Essential oil

Blend the yogurt, strawberries, and honey. Add wheat bran and lavender essential oil. Massage scrub gently to wet body. Rinse.

BATH FIZZES
&
BATH POWDERS

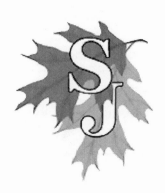

CR

Baking Soda, Citric Acid and Essential Oil

1 cup Baking Soda
½ cup Citric Acid
Essential Oil
1 teaspoon Water
Plastic molds (ice cube trays/candy molds etc.)

Blend baking soda and citric acid well in a bowl. In a separate bowl mix water and a few drops of essential oil. Mix dry and wet ingredients together until crumbly. Quickly fill molds with ingredients. Let sit over 12-24 hours. When dry remove fizzies from molds and store in an airtight container. Use one or two in bath.

NOTE: Don't add too much witch hazel or the fizzies will start foaming.

CRCRCRCRCRCRCRCRCRCRCRCRCRCRCRCRCRCRCRCRCRCRCR

Baking Soda, Citric Acid, Witch Hazel, Essential Oil and Turmeric

2 cups Baking Soda
1 cup Citric Acid
Witch Hazel (in a spray bottle)
10-20 drops of Citrus Essential Oils (citrus and lavender)
1 teaspoon Turmeric for color
Hard Plastic Molds

Mix baking soda, citric acid and turmeric in a bowl. Add 10-20 drops of citrus essential oil. Spray witch hazel into mixture. Mix quickly. Spray witch hazel a little at a time. Mix until mixture holds together. Place in molds. Pack tightly. Flip molds and empty the fizzies out. Let them sit for 12 hours. Once dry store in airtight container. Add one or two to bath.

ଔଔଔଔଔଔଔଔଔଔଔଔଔଔଔଔଔଔଔଔଔଔଔଔଔଔଔ

Baking Soda, Citric Acid, Witch Hazel, Essential Oil and Dried Lavender Flowers

2 cups Baking Soda
1 cup Citric Acid
Witch Hazel (in a spray bottle)
10-20 drops of Lavender Essential Oil
1 tablespoon Dried Lavender Flowers
Hard Plastic Molds

Mix baking soda, citric acid and dried lavender flowers in a bowl. Add lavender essential oil. Spray witch hazel into mixture. Mix quickly. Continue to spray witch hazel a little at a time. Mix until mixture holds together. Place mixture in molds. Pack tightly. Flip molds and empty out fizzies. Let dry 12 hours. Store in airtight container. Use one or two in bath.

ଔଔଔଔଔଔଔଔଔଔଔଔଔଔଔଔଔଔଔଔଔଔଔଔଔଔଔ

Baking Soda, Lemon Juice, Witch Hazel, and Essential Oil

½ cup Baking Soda
4 drops Essential Oil
4 drops Lemon Juice
8 Tbsp. Witch Hazel
Spray Bottle
Plastic Molds

Mix baking soda in a bowl . Mix the essential oil, lemon juice and witch hazel and put in a spray bottle. Spray liquid into the baking soda and mix. Keep adding liquid until baking soda starts to sticks together. Put in mold and pack tightly. Flip molds and remove fizzies. Let them dry 12 hours. Store in air tight container. Use one or two in bath.

Essential Oil, Baking Soda and Corn Starch

10 - 20 drops of Essential Oil
1 cup Baking Soda
1 cup Cornstarch

Mix baking soda and cornstarch. Put in a jar. Add your essential oil. Let powder sit for about 24 hours. Add to bath water.

NOTE: As you add the essential oil, shake the container to mix well and break up clumps.

❧ 7 ❧
HAIR

> *Beauty draws us with a single hair ~*
> *Alexander Pope*

ɷɷɷɷɷɷɷɷɷɷɷɷɷɷɷɷɷɷɷɷɷɷɷɷɷɷ

DRY CLEANED HAIR

I don't know about you, but if my hair isn't clean I'm miserable. I mean grouchy miserable. This got me to thinking. If the 'poo-hits-the-fan' and we don't have running water or it is weeks or longer before we can get water – how will we wash our hair? I can tell, like most of you, if I go more than a day or two without washing my hair ... well - gross!! Right? Just the thought of not washing my hair sends me back to grade school days when somehow year after year, I always ended up sitting behind that person, who was more occupied with other things than their hygiene - we're talking oil slick hair. A memory burnt into my head.

So, how do we avoid the "oil slick" hair syndrome when water is scarce or none at all? I mean really, you can only do the ponytail, bun, braid or hat thing so long before it will actually stay up on its own (don't ewww me - you know what I'm talking about.)

Well, here is what I came up with. The first thing I found was corn starch. You just work a quarter of a cup of it into your hair and brush it out. It lifts all the oil out of the hair. Just section your hair and pour a little corn starch next to the roots. Once all your hair is sectioned and the corn starch applied just kinda massage it into your scalp; pulling it up from the roots on to the hair shaft (leave it in for about 3 minutes to allow the oil to absorb). Then brush it out. This worked pretty well.

Next, Quaker Oats, not just for fiber anymore! I must admit this one would be a little tough for me, for no other reason except, I actually like to eat oatmeal. So, to me, using perfectly good food on my head - would be ... well I'm just sayin' I'd have to ponder long and hard before using this one. It's the stomach vs hair thing. But, for those of you where there would be no love lost, just apply a cup of oatmeal to your hair (oh, dry and uncooked of course) and work it through with your fingers. The oats, like the corn starch, will absorb the oil in your hair. I guess the real reason for me not trying this

ෆ෪ෆ෪ෆ෪ෆ෪ෆ෪ෆ෪ෆ෪ෆ෪ෆ෪ෆ෪ෆ෪ෆ෪ෆ෪ෆ෪ෆ෪ෆ෪ෆ෪ෆ෪

method is for fear I'd be tempted to add cinnamon and honey and begin sucking on my hair! Juuuust kidding.

Moving on. How about this? Flour? This was actually the method our forefathers, er ... probably our foremothers used. Just take a handful of flour and work it through your hair, down to the roots, with your fingertips. Afterwards, brush it out. Your hair will be clean (it may be a little whitish but clean).

And this one? Good ol' baby powder. Just sprinkle it liberally into your hair making sure to get it down into your roots and then brush it out. (I've used baby powder in a pinch before. It did work great, it just made my hair smell like ... well a baby's hiney all day.)

And lastly, baking soda. As you may know, baking soda has a variety of uses and quite possibly is one of the items you already have packed in your emergency bag and pantry. Like with the others items, just sprinkle some baking soda in your hair and work it in to remove all the oils. Then brush it out.

As you will note, each of the items mentioned has a common theme - they all are a powder form, well with the exception of the oats. If you are thinking to yourself, 'this just isn't for me', never fear, there are actually dry hair products out on the market you may want to look into. But before you get too caught up into looking, think about this, in an "end of the world as we know it" world you will not be able to replace the hair product if purchased, so, it may behoove you to get used to what items will actually be available.

Knowing you have a way to make yourself feel a little better physically in a time of crisis could be a huge morale boaster. Just sayin'.

SCALP
TREATMENTS

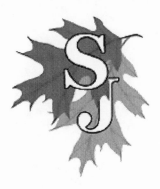

ଔଔଔଔଔଔଔଔଔଔଔଔଔଔଔଔଔଔଔଔଔଔଔଔଔଔଔ

Essential Oils/Carrier Oils
for Hair Type

Normal Hair
Essential Oils: Lavender and Rosemary.
Carrier Oils: Coconut, Jojoba and Sweet Almond.

Dry Hair:
Essential Oils: Lavender, Rose hip, Rosemary, and Sandalwood.
Carrier Oils: Coconut, Jojoba, Sesame and Sweet Almond.

Fine Hair:
Essential Oils: Geranium, Lavender, and Rosemary.
Carrier Oils: Olive and Sesame.

Damaged/Chemically Treated Hair:
Essential Oils: Geranium, Lavender, Rosemary, and Sandalwood.
Carrier Oils: Coconut, Jojoba, Sesame and Sweet Almond.

Dry Scalp/Dandruff:
Essential Oils: Eucalyptus, Geranium Lavender, and Rosemary.
Carrier Oils: Coconut , Jojoba, Olive, and Sweet Almond.

ෆෆෆෆෆෆෆෆෆෆෆෆෆෆෆෆෆෆෆෆෆෆෆෆෆෆ

Apple Cider Vinegar

Apple Cider Vinegar
Water

Take spray bottle and mix half water and half apple cider vinegar in the bottle. Spray on your scalp and let sit for 15 minutes each time before washing your hair.

ෆෆෆෆෆෆෆෆෆෆෆෆෆෆෆෆෆෆෆෆෆෆෆෆෆෆ

Tea Tree Oil and Olive Oil

2 drops Tea Tree Oil
1 tablespoon Olive Oil

Combine one tablespoon of olive oil and two drops of tea tree oil. Massage the solution all over your scalp. Wash out.

NOTE: Tea tree oil is naturally antibacterial and antifungal. It kills microbes that cause dry, itchy scalp.

ෆෆෆෆෆෆෆෆෆෆෆෆෆෆෆෆෆෆෆෆෆෆෆෆෆෆ

Baking Soda

1-2 tablespoons Baking Soda
Water

Mix baking soda with small amounts of water to make a thick paste. Massage into damp hair. Let sit for 15 minutes. Rinse with water, then shampoo hair.

NOTE: Sodium bicarbonate (baking soda) breaks down anything acidic.

CRUR

Lemon Juice/Olive Oil

2 tablespoons Lemon Juice
2 tablespoons Olive Oil

Mix lemon juice and olive oil together. Massage into damp scalp. Let mixture sit for 20 minutes. Rinse and shampoo hair.

CRURURURURURURURURURURURURURURURURURURURURURURUR

Cornmeal/Cornstarch

1 tablespoon Cornmeal (or cornstarch)

Pour cornmeal or cornstarch into a shaker type container. Sprinkle cornmeal onto dry hair and scalp. Leave on for 10 minutes. Brush cornmeal out completely.

NOTE: Cornmeal or cornstarch is an inexpensive way to remove oil and grease from hair.

CRURURURURURURURURURURURURURURURURURURURURURURUR

DANDRUFF
TREATMENTS

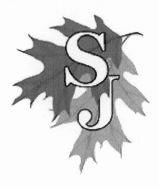

ೞೞೞೞೞೞೞೞೞೞೞೞೞೞೞೞೞೞೞೞೞೞೞೞೞ

Aspirin

2 Aspirin
Shampoo

Crush aspirin into fine powder. Add aspirin to your normal amount of shampoo. Wash hair and leave shampoo in for 1-2 minutes. Rinse well.

ೞೞೞೞೞೞೞೞೞೞೞೞೞೞೞೞೞೞೞೞೞೞೞೞೞ

Baking Soda

Baking Soda

Wet hair. Apply a handful of baking soda into your scalp and rub vigorously. Rinse thoroughly (no shampoo)

ೞೞೞೞೞೞೞೞೞೞೞೞೞೞೞೞೞೞೞೞೞೞೞೞೞ

Lemon Juice

2 tablespoons and 1 teaspoon Lemon Juice
1 cup water

Massage 2 tablespoons of lemon juice onto your scalp. Rinse with water. Then add 1 teaspoon of lemon juice into 1 cup of water and rinse hair with it.

ೞೞೞೞೞೞೞೞೞೞೞೞೞೞೞೞೞೞೞೞೞೞೞೞೞ

Mouthwash

Mouthwash (Alcohol-based)

Wash hair. Rinse with mouthwash. Follow with regular conditioner.

CR

Salt

Salt

Shake salt onto a dry scalp and massage gently. Shampoo hair.

CRCRCRCRCRCRCRCRCRCRCRCRCRCRCRCRCRCRCRCRCRCRCRCRCRCR

Apple Cider Vinegar

2 cups Apple Cider Vinegar
2 cups Cold Water

After shampooing rinse hair with apple cider vinegar mixed with cold water.

CRCRCRCRCRCRCRCRCRCRCRCRCRCRCRCRCRCRCRCRCRCRCRCRCRCR

Olive Oil

¼ teaspoon Olive Oil

Warm olive oil. Apply to scalp in circular motions before going to bed. Wash hair with a mild shampoo in the morning.

CRCRCRCRCRCRCRCRCRCRCRCRCRCRCRCRCRCRCRCRCRCRCRCRCRCR

A luke warm oil head-massage is considered one of the best home remedy to get rid of dandruff.

CRCRCRCRCRCRCRCRCRCRCRCRCRCRCRCRCRCRCRCRCRCRCRCRCRCR

രു

Lemon Juice and Coconut Oil

1 tablespoon Lemon Juice
5 tablespoons Coconut Oil

Blend lemon juice with coconut oil. Apply to the scalp. Leave for 20 to 30 minutes. Wash with a shampoo.

രു

Aloe Vera Gel

Aloe Vera Gel

Apply aloe vera gel to scalp. Leave on 15 minutes. Rinse out.

രു

Aloe vera gel fights dandruff and eliminates dandruff flakes so the scalp can heal

രു

Eggs

2 Eggs

Beat eggs. Apply to scalp. Leave on for 1 hour. Rinse.

രു

ෲෲෲෲෲෲෲෲෲෲෲෲෲෲෲෲෲෲෲෲෲෲෲෲෲ

Almond Oil (Coconut Oil or Olive Oil)

1 teaspoon Almond Oil (or other oil)

Warm almond oil. Massage on scalp. Leave on overnight. Rinse.

ෲෲෲෲෲෲෲෲෲෲෲෲෲෲෲෲෲෲෲෲෲෲෲෲෲ

Onion

Onion
Lemon Juice

Crush an onion into a paste. Apply the paste to your scalp. Leave it on for one hour. Wash thoroughly. Apply lemon juice to remove smell of onion from your hair.

ෲෲෲෲෲෲෲෲෲෲෲෲෲෲෲෲෲෲෲෲෲෲෲෲෲ

Soap Nut

Soap Nuts

Crush soap nuts into powder. Add water to make a paste. Apply to scalp and leave on 2 hours. Rinse.

ෲෲෲෲෲෲෲෲෲෲෲෲෲෲෲෲෲෲෲෲෲෲෲෲෲ

Apple Juice

2 tablespoons Apple Juice
Water

Mix apple juice and water. Apply to scalp. Leave on 5 to 10 minutes. Wash hair.

149

> **Apples have enzymes that eliminate dead skin cells that cause scalp flakes**

Tea Tree Oil

Apply a few drops of tea tree oil to the scalp and massage in.

Lemon and Garlic

1 tablespoon Lemon Juice
2 tablespoon Garlic

Mix lemon juice and garlic and make a paste. Apply to scalp. Leave on 20 to 30 minutes. Shampoo hair.

NOTE: Garlic is a natural antibiotic and kills bacteria on scalp.

Rosemary Oil and Coconut Oil

¼ teaspoon Rosemary Oil
¼ teaspoon Coconut Oil

Mix rosemary oil and coconut oil. Apply to your scalp.

ෆෲෆෲෆෲෆෲෆෲෆෲෆෲෆෲෆෲෆෲෆෲෆෲෆෲෆෲෆෲ

HOT OIL
TREATMENTS

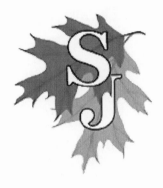

Oils for Hot Hair Treatments

Avocado Oil - One of the most moisturizing oils. Good for dry hair.

Castor Oil - Heavier oil. Seals in moisture. Great for oily hair. Helps thicken and strength hair.

Coconut Oil - Light and non-greasy. All hair types. Penetrates hair shaft. Good for flaking or dandruff.

Grape Seed Oil - All hair types. Light. Moisturizing. Natural heat protectant. Hair strengthener. Good for dry scalp and dandruff.

Jojoba Oil - Good for oily hair. Leaves hair soft and light

Olive Oil - Seals in moisture.

Tea Tree Oil - Unclogs hair follicles. Eliminates dandruff. Moisturizes hair and scalp.

Safflower Oil - Moisturizes hair. Stimulates blood circulation. Promote hair growth and thickness. Good for dry chemically treated hair.

Sesame Oil – All hair types. Adds shine. Used to slow hair loss and treat thinning hair.

Grape Seed Oil and Aloe Vera Gel

2 tablespoons Grape Seed Oil
½ cup Aloe Vera Gel
½ Water

Mix grape seed oil, aloe vera gel, and water. Apply to ends of your hair just before using a hair dryer or flat iron.

Coconut Oil and Olive Oil

2 tablespoons Coconut Oil
1 tablespoon Olive Oil (optional)
1 tablespoon Jojoba Oil (optional)
1 cup Water

Begin with wet hair. Boil water. Turn off heat. Place coconut oil in glass container (mix olive oil or Jojoba oil – optional). Place container in water to warm coconut oil. Using your fingers, dip into the oil and massage into hair from scalp to roots using all the oil. Wrap hair in towel, Saran Wrap, a plastic shower cap or even a plastic grocery bag. Leave from 20 minutes. Wash and rinse.

NOTE: Jojoba oil is a natural fungicide

Olive Oil, Coconut Oil and Honey

2 tablespoons Olive Oil
2 tablespoons Coconut Oil
1 tablespoon Honey
1 cup Water

Boil water in saucepan. Remove from heat. Add olive oil, coconut oil and honey in a glass bowl or mug. Place bowl in saucepan of water to heat. Once ingredients melted apply to dry hair. Wrap hair in plastic wrap or a shower cap. Leave on overnight or as long as you can. Wash and rinse.

NOTE: Olive oil is good for a dry scalp

Coconut Oil, Jojoba Oil and Essential Oil

8 tablespoons Coconut Oil
4 tablespoon Jojoba Oil (or Olive Oil)
15-20 drops Tea Tree Oil

Place coconut oil in a bowl and soften. Add jojoba oil and essential oil and make cream. Put in jar with lid. Add to wet hair. Cover with plastic wrap/shower cap/plastic grocery bag. Leave on for 30 minute. Shampoo.

Almond Oil, Avocado Oil and Olive Oil

½ cup Almond Oil
¼ cup Avocado Oil
¼ cup Olive Oil
1 cup Water

Boil water in saucepan. Remove from heat. In a glass mug/jar mix ingredients. Sit the jar in saucepan. Heat until warm (not hot) Apply to damp hair. Apply plastic wrap/a plastic grocery bag/shower cap over your hair. Cover with a towel. Leave on for 20 minutes. Shampoo.

CR

Soybean Oil, Sandalwood Oil, Geranium Oil and Lavender Oil

½ cup of Soybean Oil
8 drops of Sandalwood Oil
8 drops of Geranium Oil
8 drops of Lavender Oil
1 cup Water

Heat water in a saucepan to boiling. Remove from heat. Mix ingredients in a glass jar/mug. Place jar in saucepan and heat mixture. Apply to damp hair. Apply plastic wrap/shower cap/plastic grocery bag. Leave on for 20 minutes. Shampoo.

CRCRCRCRCRCRCRCRCRCRCRCRCRCRCRCRCRCRCRCRCRCRCRCR

HAIRSPRAYS

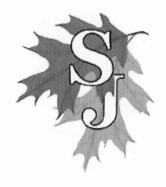

CR

Aloe Vera Gel

½ cup Aloe Vera Gel
½ cup Distilled Water

Mix aloe vera gel and distilled water. Place in a spray-type bottle. Spray hair as needed to prevent dry frizzy hair.

NOTE: Aloe vera gel pulls moisture from the air to keep hair smooth.

CRCRCRCRCRCRCRCRCRCRCRCRCRCRCRCRCRCRCRCRCRCRCRCR

White Sugar, Vodka
and Essential Oil

1 ½ cups Water
2 tablespoons White Sugar
1 tablespoon Vodka (80 proof or 100 proof)
10-15 drops of Essential Oil

Boil water. Remove from heat and add sugar. Once sugar is dissolved allow to cool. Add alcohol and essential oils. Put in a spray bottle. Spray hair. Let dry. Repeat.

CRCRCRCRCRCRCRCRCRCRCRCRCRCRCRCRCRCRCRCRCRCRCRCR

Maple Syrup, Rubbing Alcohol and Essential Oil

½ cup Water
2 teaspoons Maple Syrup
2 tablespoons Rubbing Alcohol
8 drops Essential Oil

Boil water. Remove from heat. Add maple syrup. Add alcohol and oil. Cool. Pour into spray- type bottle. Spray hair. Let dry. Repeat.

Sugar and Essential Oil

1 cup Water
4 teaspoons Sugar
6-8 drops Essential Oil

Heat water in small saucepan to boiling. Add sugar. Stir to dissolve. Cool. Add essential oil. Pour in spray bottle. Spray hair. Let dry. Repeat.

Lemon (Orange), Rubbing Alcohol and Essential Oil

1 Lemon (for Light Hair
1 Orange (for Dark Hair)
2 cups Water
Essential Oil
1 tablespoon Rubbing Alcohol

Slice the lemon into wedges. Place wedges in a pot of water and boil down to one cup of liquid. Cool. Add essential oil and alcohol. Pour liquid into spray bottle. Spray hair. Let dry. Repeat.

SHAMPOO

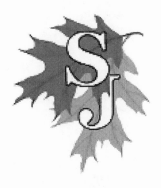

CR

Baking Soda

2 tablespoons Baking Soda
2 cups Water

Mix baking soda and water. Pour the mixture through hair and work through hair. Rinse.

NOTE: For the best hair ever, follow up with 2 tablespoons of apple cider vinegar and 2 cups of water.

CRCRCRCRCRCRCRCRCRCRCRCRCRCRCRCRCRCRCRCRCRCRCR

Castile Soap

1 tablespoon Castile Soap
3 tablespoon Water

Mix castile soap with water and shampoo hair. Rinse.

CRCRCRCRCRCRCRCRCRCRCRCRCRCRCRCRCRCRCRCRCRCRCR

Castile Soap and Jojoba Oil

¼ cup Water
¼ cup liquid Castile Soap
½ teaspoon Jojoba (or other Vegetable Oil)
Few drops of Peppermint Oil
Few drops of Tea Tree Oil

Mix all ingredients. Store in a spray bottle. Shake before use. Spray on wet hair and shampoo.

CRCRCRCRCRCRCRCRCRCRCRCRCRCRCRCRCRCRCRCRCRCRCR

Coconut Milk, Castile Soap, and Vitamin E

¼ cup Coconut Milk
1/3 cup Liquid Castile Soap
1 teaspoon Vitamin E (or olive oil or almond oil)
10 to 20 drops of essential oils

Combine all ingredients. Put in bottle or jar. Shake well to mix. Apply to wet hair and shampoo hair. Rinse.

ೞೞೞೞೞೞೞೞೞೞೞೞೞೞೞೞೞೞೞೞೞೞೞೞ

HAIR CONDITIONERS

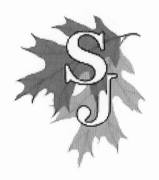

ഇരഇരഇരഇരഇരഇരഇരഇരഇരഇരഇരഇരഇരഇരഇരഇരഇര

GOING BANANAS

I overheard someone say bananas were nature's secret to repairing and preserving beautiful hair. I thought to myself, "Hmmm I wonder...?" And, with curiosity getting the best of me I decided to do a little research on what the benefits of bananas were and if they really could be used as hair conditioner.

What I found was that bananas are loaded with vitamins A, B, C and E and potassium. They also contain tryptophan; which is a rich amino acid, and potassium. And, as an added benefit they are rich in natural oils and carbohydrates. Good news so far!

The vitamins and minerals contained in bananas are supposed to bring out the natural elasticity of the hair, add super softening properties to the hair shaft and prevents split ends. Wow! Bananas would be perfect for dry, brittle, sun-damaged, heat-damaged, and dyed hair. Sounds like a commercial for those expensive conditioners, right? Well, less all the chemically stuff added. We may just have a winner! But the true test would be how well it really worked.

I drug out a bowl and fork and retrieve a banana from its resting place in the fruit bowl. I washed my hair and left it damp as I prepared my banana delight; mashing the banana up in the bowl to make a "banana paste". Then over the sink, I put the paste in my hair and put on a cheap shower cap (you can also wrapped your hair with plastic wrap or a plastic grocery bag – the key here is to keep the heat in). Then I left the mixture on for about an hour.

This is not the only way to make a banana conditioner. You can also take a bananas and mash it up with ¼ cup of honey. Or, a banana and a ¼ cup of olive oil and an egg white. There are lots of variations. Have fun and experiment.

For me, being a girl who hasn't the patience nor time for a lot of hoopla, I opted for the 'lone' banana mixture. Let me stress, you want to make sure you really, really, really mash the banana up well – like pudding really well - or you will find yourself picking banana

ωεωεωεωεωεωεωεωεωεωεωεωεωεωεωεωεωεωεωεωεωε

pieces-parts out of your hair over the sink! Yep, that was me. Just consider this as me taking the hit for you. Just sayin'. After the pieces were removed, it was the time of reckoning. I rinsed the mixture out of my hair ... and wow! Where have you been all my life?? My hair was soooo soft. And when my hair dried it looked fantastic!

Now happily, that bunch of bananas that usually just sits in the fruit bowl begging for attention now has a special purpose!

Chalk one up for survival hair treatments!

Castor Oil, Malt Vinegar, Glycerin, Herbal Oil, and Shampoo

1 teaspoon Castor Oil
1 teaspoon Malt Vinegar
1 teaspoon Glycerin
1 teaspoon Herbal Oil
1 teaspoon Shampoo

Mix castor oil, malt vinegar, glycerin, herbal oil, and shampoo. Apply the mixture to hair. Leave on 20 minutes. Shampoo out.

Onions and Cabbage

Onion
Cabbage
Essential Oil

Grate onions and cabbage. Let sit overnight. Add few drops essential oil. Apply the mixture to your hair. Leave in 20 minutes. Shampoo out.

NOTE: Use an essential oil of your choice to counter the smell of onions

Henna Powder and Yogurt

Henna Powder
2 tablespoon Plain Yogurt
Pinch Sugar

Mix henna powder, plain yogurt and sugar. Make a paste. Apply to hair. Leave on 20 minutes. Rinse.

CR

NOTE: Henna Powder and Yogurt is a good combination for Oily Hair.

CRCRCRCRCRCRCRCRCRCRCRCRCRCRCRCRCRCRCRCRCRCRCRCRCR

Henna and Olive Oil

Henna
1 tablespoon Olive Oil
Milk (warm)

Mix henna with olive oil. Add enough warm milk to make a paste. Leave on for 20 minutes. Rinse.

CRCRCRCRCRCRCRCRCRCRCRCRCRCRCRCRCRCRCRCRCRCRCRCRCR

Gelatin

1 teaspoon Gelatin
Water

Mix gelatin and water. Pour on to hair. Towel dry hair.

CRCRCRCRCRCRCRCRCRCRCRCRCRCRCRCRCRCRCRCRCRCRCRCRCR

Aloe Vera and Coconut Oil

¼ cup Aloe Vera Gel
¼ cup Coconut Oil
1 cup water

Bring water to a light simmer. Combine aloe vera and coconut oil in glass mug/jar. Sit jar down in water until coconut oil is melted. Mix to make a creamy paste. Apply to clean hair. Leave on 15 minutes. Shampoo hair.

ରେ ରେ ରେ ରେ ରେ ରେ ରେ ରେ ରେ ରେ ରେ ରେ ରେ ରେ ରେ ରେ

NOTE: Coconut oil is rich in fatty acids to help restore and moisturize your hair.

ରେ ରେ ରେ ରେ ରେ ରେ ରେ ରେ ରେ ରେ ରେ ରେ ରେ ରେ ରେ ରେ

Raw Eggs

1 Egg

Apply egg mixture to scalp. Leave on for 20 minutes. Shampoo hair.

NOTE: For normal hair: use entire egg. For oily hair use egg whites. For dry hair use egg yolks.

ରେ ରେ ରେ ରେ ରେ ରେ ରେ ରେ ରେ ରେ ରେ ରେ ରେ ରେ ରେ ରେ

Honey and Olive Oil

½ cup Honey
1-2 tablespoons Olive Oil

Combine honey and olive oil. Massage into clean, damp hair. Leave on for 20 minutes. Rinse.

ରେ ରେ ରେ ରେ ରେ ରେ ରେ ରେ ରେ ରେ ରେ ରେ ରେ ରେ ରେ ରେ

Apple Cider Vinegar

½ cup Apple Cider Vinegar
2 cups Water

Mix water and apple cider vinegar. Put in spray type bottle. Spray on damp hair. Rinse well.

NOTE: One of my favorite conditioners!!

CR

Egg and Olive Oil

2 Eggs
3 tablespoons Olive Oil
Essential Oils (Optional)

Combine eggs and olive oil. Add essential oil. Apply to hair. Wrap hair plastic wrap/shower cap/plastic grocery bag. Leave on for 30 minutes. Rinse.

NOTE: Olive Oil and Eggs good for Dry Hair.

CRCRCRCRCRCRCRCRCRCRCRCRCRCRCRCRCRCRCRCRCRCRCRCRCRCR

Cucumber and Egg

¼ Cucumber
Egg
2 tablespoon Olive Oil

Peel cucumber. Mix egg, olive oil and cucumber into a paste. Massage into hair. Leave on for 10 minutes. Rinse thoroughly.

CRCRCRCRCRCRCRCRCRCRCRCRCRCRCRCRCRCRCRCRCRCRCRCRCRCR

> The protein in an egg yolk will make hair strands strong.

CRCRCRCRCRCRCRCRCRCRCRCRCRCRCRCRCRCRCRCRCRCRCRCRCRCR

Avocado

Avocado
Essential Oil (optional)

CR

Mash an avocado into a paste. Add a couple of drops of essential oil. Massage into hair. Leave on for 20 minutes. Shampoo.

CRCRCRCRCRCRCRCRCRCRCRCRCRCRCRCRCRCRCRCRCRCRCRCRCR

Mayonnaise

2 tablespoons Mayonnaise

Massaging mayonnaise into scalp. Wrap hair in plastic wrap/shower cap/plastic grocery bag. Leave on for 20 minutes. Shampoo.

CRCRCRCRCRCRCRCRCRCRCRCRCRCRCRCRCRCRCRCRCRCRCRCRCR

Vegetable Oil

1 tablespoon Vegetable Oil

Massage vegetable oil into hair. Wrap hair in plastic wrap/shower cap/plastic grocery bag. Leave on one hour. Shampoo.

CRCRCRCRCRCRCRCRCRCRCRCRCRCRCRCRCRCRCRCRCRCRCRCRCR

Rosemary, Apple Cider Vinegar and Essential Oil

1 cup apple cider vinegar
2 tablespoons fresh or dried rosemary
10 drops Essential oil

Heat the vinegar to simmering. Add rosemary. Cover and steep for 2 hours. Strain. Add essential oil to liquid. Pour in bottle or jar. Add 2 tablespoons of the mixture to 1 cup of water and massage through your hair after shampooing. Rinse well.

CRCRCRCRCRCRCRCRCRCRCRCRCRCRCRCRCRCRCRCRCRCRCRCRCR

HAIR COLOR

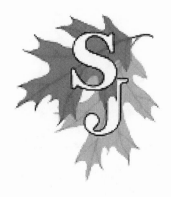

CℛCℛCℛCℛCℛCℛCℛCℛCℛCℛCℛCℛCℛCℛCℛCℛCℛCℛCℛCℛCℛCℛCℛ

Golden Hair Color

Saffron and Lemon Juice

2 cups Water
Large pinch Saffron threads
1 tablespoon Lemon Juice

Boil water. Place saffron threads into a large bowl. Pour water over the saffron. Let soak for 15 minutes. In sieve, strain out saffron. Add lemon juice to liquid. Over the bowl, pour liquid through hair recapturing the liquid. Repeat 15-20 times. On last rinse leave in hair for 15 minutes. Rinse.

CℛCℛCℛCℛCℛCℛCℛCℛCℛCℛCℛCℛCℛCℛCℛCℛCℛCℛCℛCℛCℛCℛCℛ

Blonde Highlights/Brightener

Calendula Petals, Chamomile Flowers
Lemon Peel and Apple Cider Vinegar

2 cups Water
3 tablespoons Dried Calendula Petals
3 tablespoons Chamomile Flowers
3 tablespoons Chopped Lemon Peel
2 tablespoons Apple Cider Vinegar

Boil water. Add dried calendula petals, chamomile flowers and lemon peel. Remove from the heat. Let steep 3 hours. Strain out the herbs using a sieve. Add apple cider vinegar. Pour into bottle. Pour over your hair. Massage gently into your scalp and rinse.

CℛCℛCℛCℛCℛCℛCℛCℛCℛCℛCℛCℛCℛCℛCℛCℛCℛCℛCℛCℛCℛCℛCℛ

171

Red – Gold Highlight Hair Color

Crushed Marigold Flower and Red Wine

1/3 cup Crushed Marigold Flowers (or 3 tablespoons Dried Calendula Petals)
1 ½ cups Water
¼ cup Red Wine

Heat water to simmer. Add marigold flowers (or dried calendula petals). Simmer 20 minutes. Remove from heat. Cool. Strain to remove marigold flowers. Add red wine to the liquid and put in large bowl. Over the bowl, pour liquid through hair recapturing the liquid. Repeat several times. Allow your hair to dry naturally in the sun if possible.

NOTE: Repeat this process every time you wash your hair until you're happy with the color.

CRQRQRQRQRQRQRQRQRQRQRQRQRQRQRQRQRQRQRQRQR

Rich Brown Tones

Walnut Shells OR Black Tea, Cherry Tree Bark, Whole Cloves

1/3 cup Walnut Shells (or black tea, cherry tree bark, whole cloves)
2 ½ cups Water

Heat water to a simmer. Simmer walnut shells (or black tea, cherry tree bark or whole cloves) for 20 minutes. Remove from heat. Cool. Strain out herbs. When cooled, strain out the herbs. Place liquid in large bowl. Over the bowl, pour liquid through hair recapturing the liquid. Repeat several times. Allow your hair to dry naturally. Do this every time you wash your hair until you reach the desired shade.

CRQRQRQRQRQRQRQRQRQRQRQRQRQRQRQRQRQRQRQRQR

CR

Very Dark Brown/Black

Black Walnut Powder

¼ cup Black Walnut Powder
3 cups Water

Place water in quart mason jar. Place black walnut powder in cheesecloth bag. Steep mason jar for at least 6 hours or overnight. After shampooing, use as a rinse . Dry in the sun. Repeat daily or as needed to darken and maintain dark shade.

NOTE: Black walnut powder will create very dark hair.

NOTE: Black walnut powder will provide the darkest coverage for grey hair. Repeat daily or as needed to darken and maintain dark shade.

CRCRCRCRCRCRCRCRCRCRCRCRCRCRCRCRCRCRCRCRCRCRCRCR

Dark Brown

Coffee Granule and Hot Coffee

1 tablespoon Instant Coffee Granules
¼ cup of Instant Hot Coffee (or brewed hot coffee)
½ cup hair conditioner

Pour conditioner into a cup. Add instant coffee granules. Mix together until thoroughly mixed. Add hot coffee to the conditioner/coffee mix . Let sit for five minutes. Apply small amounts at a time to dry hair. Continue until all hair is covered. Massage for two minutes. Wrap hair in plastic wrap/shower cap/plastic grocery bag. Leave on 30 minutes. Rinse and shampoo hair.

❧ 8 ❧
HYGIENE

> *Take care of your body.*
> *It's the only place you*
> *have to live. –*
> *Jim Rohn*

CR

OIL PULLING? HOW DO YOU PULL OIL?

I am always on a quest to replace, substitute or find something I can use in lieu of any - item, tool or food - that I won't be able to get or have access to when the poo-hits-the-fan, and this holds true for health and medicinal items as well.

It's a given, prevention is better than a cure but who has the time for all this prevention stuff, right? But, prevention just screams of sacrifice or more work than we care to do, right?. If we can't buy it to do it for us, we won't have anything to do with it or ...if it's not fast and painless, forget about it.

What I've learned by living pretty close to off the-grid is that it forces you to "make do" with what you have on hand - something we all need to do a little more practicing on – because if and, when the poo ever hits the fan it will be second nature.

I'm not a "greenie-naturey" type of person (no disrespect or offense to those of you who are), but I know that when the poo hits the fan we will have to rely on the things in our gardens, herbs and spices along with our food stores and pantries as major sources for anything and everything that ails us - which all leads up to my point in all of this.

I was chewing on a piece of soft buttery garlic crust from my homemade Friday-night pizza one ... well Friday night, when I felt this oddness on one of my back molars. I spit the bite of crust out on the kitchen counter (I know, ewwww) and raced to the bathroom mirror, only to learn I had broken a porcelain crown – a piece of it at least - the front portion ... yep the part exposed to the outside world was gone – with the back portion securely in place. Panicked, I dug through my partially eating pizza bite still sitting on the kitchen counter in hopes of retrieving the missing piece of porcelain (go with me – I was desperate!) all the while not really sure what I would do with it once it was found. Denied - I had eaten it. And, no, I didn't consider waiting for the alternative ...don't even go there (no pun intended.)

175

ೂೞೂೞೂೞೂೞೂೞೂೞೂೞೂೞೂೞೂೞೂೞೂೞೂೞೂೞೂೞೂೞೂೞೂೞ

My first thought ..."It's Friday night and I have two long days before I could even hope to see the light of a dentist's office ... that is, if I could even get an appointment on Monday. My mind began to race "what would I do if this had occurred in a poo-hits-the-fan scenario where there was no dentist?" I do this type of thinking a lot by the way - the what-if's.

Immediately I got on my computer to search the internet for something I could do in the meantime to prevent any bacteria build up - secretly hoping for some sort of miracle tooth regrowth, just sayin'.

While in my search; as also happens a lot, I got a little side-tracked from my initial query of something to keep my teeth free of bacteria until I could get to a dentist, when I stumbled upon ...oil pulling. I know this is going to sound kinda oxymoron-ish. How can you pull oil? Well intrigue set in and I abandoned my initial search for this new found intriguement.

Oil pulling is nothing new, I mean really nothing new. In fact it is an old Ayurvedic medicinal practice that evolved in India thousands of years ago. "Hmmm." I thought to myself. "If the Avurvedic did this ... and people are still doing it, it must be natural and healthy."

As most know, just about all the medicines out there today, originally began as natural ingredients. Then colorings, chemicals and additives began to be added and who knows what we're using now.

So what is oil pulling? (Caveat: This is going to sound really weird – I mean really weird.) By taking a tablespoon of vegetable based oil; such as sun flower oil, sesame seed oil, safflower oil, coconut oil, et cetera and swishing it around in your mouth for 20 minutes, the oil acts as a detoxifier. As you work the oil around your teeth and gums while swishing, it "pulls" out bacteria and other bad stuff from your body. The reason for the 20 minutes is it is long enough to break down the plaque and bacteria but not long enough for the body to reabsorb the toxins and bacteria back into your system - or so I understand.

CR

Now, I know you are probably thinking, "20 minutes!" I did too. But if you "pull" while taking a shower, checking your emails, or even fixing breakfast, I promise the time will be over before you even notice.

I tried it - that very next morning - with coconut oil (which is not oil at first but hold it under your tongue or chew it and you'll have your oil.) I was really surprised at the results. My teeth, which I'm a little anal about, felt really clean. Like dental visit cleaning, clean.

While you are "pulling" the oil will become thicker. When you finally spit it out (NOT in the sink or toilet by the way ... we are talking oil here), it becomes kinda white and foamy – if it did not you didn't swish long enough. I rinsed my mouth out with warm salt water and brush my teeth with baking soda and peroxide. I personally have found that mornings are good for me because you are supposed to do oil pulling on an empty stomach. Some actually do it up to three times a day.

Let's face it, our mouths are the gateway to all kinds of bacteria and toxins; including candida that causes gum disease and tooth decay and contributes to many other health problems, so it would only make sense to rid bacteria from the same place (remember I was initially looking for options to keep my teeth bacteria free when I stumbled on oil-pulling.)

When doing your own research; which I always encourage you doing, you will find that oil-pulling is tied to some remarkable "cures" after detoxing your body of toxins Here are just a few of oil-pulling benefits:

    Migraine headache relief
    Correcting hormone imbalances
    Reducing inflammation of arthritis
    May help with gastroenteritis
    Aids in the reduction of eczema
    May reduce symptoms of bronchitis
    Helps support normal kidney function

ख़

May help reduce sinus congestion
Some people report improved vision
Helps reduce insomnia
Reduced hangover after alcohol consumption
Aids in reducing pain
Reduces the symptoms of allergies
Helps detoxify the body of harmful metals and organisms
(Oilpulling.com)

Fortunately, I'm pretty healthy and can't report on being able to leap any tall building in a single bound or anything like that since my initial oil-pulling experience, but I will tell you my skin is softer, my hair, eyebrows and eyelashes are thicker and I have the pinkest tongue in the whole world *grin* okay maybe not in the world, but it's pretty healthy looking. And why is that a big deal? Well, have you noticed how when you have a doctor visit he/she asks you to stick out your tongue? Well, it's because the tongue can reveal a lot about your overall state of health.

So why am I even talking about oil-pulling? Well, I think that this could be a very inexpensive way to keep your mouth clean when the poo-hits-the-fan. We may no longer have access to store bought toothpaste, but it is amazing what a tablespoon of vegetable oil, some baking soda and peroxide can do to keep your mouth germ free and therefore our bodies healthier by ridding all those nasty toxins.

Oh, and when I finally got to see a dentist, he was amazed at how clean and healthy my teeth, gums and tongue were (I didn't tell him my little secret.) Just sayin'.

SHAVING CREAMS

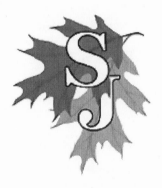

CR

Shea Butter, Coconut Oil, Rosemary Essential Oil and Peppermint Essential Oil

1/3 Shea Butter
1/3 Extra Virgin Coconut Oil
¼ Jojoba (or Almond Oil)
10 drops Rosemary Essential Oil
3-5 drops Peppermint Essential Oil

In a saucepan, combine shea butter and coconut oil. Heat over low heat. Remove from heat. Pour into glass bowl. Stir in jojoba, rosemary essential oil and peppermint essential oil. Put in cool place to solidify. Mix into a cream. Place in jar. Keep in cool dry place.

CRCRCRCRCRCRCRCRCRCRCRCRCRCRCRCRCRCRCRCRCRCRCRCR

Sunflower Oil and Glycerin Soap

¼ cup Glycerin Soap
½ teaspoon Sunflower Oil

Cut glycerin soap into chunks. Place in saucepan. Heat on low until glycerin soap melted. Add in sunflower oil. Pour mixture into a jar. Keep in cool dry place.

CRCRCRCRCRCRCRCRCRCRCRCRCRCRCRCRCRCRCRCRCRCRCRCR

Coconut Oil, Shea Butter and Olive Oil

1/3 cup Shea Butter
1/3 cup Coconut Oil
¼ cup Olive Oil

In saucepan on low, melt shea butter and coconut oil. Remove from heat. Add olive oil. Pour into a bottle or jar. Put in cool place to solidify. Mix into cream. Keep in cool dry place.

CR

Cocoa Butter, Almond Oil, Baking Soda
and Castile Soap

2 tablespoons Cocoa Butter
4 tablespoons Almond Oil
1 ½ cups Water
4 tablespoons Castile Soap
1 teaspoon Baking Soda

In small saucepan on low, heat cocoa butter and almond. Remove from heat and cool. In another saucepan heat water on low. Add castile soap and baking soda. Stir until dissolved. Mix castile soap mixture in with cocoa butter mixture. Mixed until it foams. Place in a container. Keep in cool dry place.

CRCRCRCRCRCRCRCRCRCRCRCRCRCRCRCRCRCRCRCRCRCRCRCR

Rose Water, Cocoa Butter, Glycerin, Grapeseed Oil
and Castile Soap

4 tablespoons Liquid Castille Soap
2 tablespoons Rose Water
1 tablespoon Cocoa Butter
1 tablespoon Castor Oil
1 tablespoon Grapeseed Oil
2 tablespoons Vegetable Glycerin

In saucepan melt coco butter. Remove from heat. Add castor oil and grape seed oil. Add castille soap and rose water, and then vegetable glycerin. Make into a cream. Put in jar with lid. Keep in cool dry place.

CRCRCRCRCRCRCRCRCRCRCRCRCRCRCRCRCRCRCRCRCRCRCRCR

181

രാ

Almond Oil, Beeswax, Water,
and Castile Soap

2 oz Almond Oil
½ oz Beeswax
4 oz Water
1 oz Glycerin
2 oz Liquid Castile Soap
1 teaspoon Borax
1/3 oz Grapefruit Seed Extract
20 drops Essential Oil

In saucepan over low heat melt beeswax and almond oil. Remove from heat. Add water, castile soap, glycerin, and borax. Make into a cream. Add grapefruit seed extract and essential oil. Put in jar with lid. Keep in cool dry place.

രാ

Apricot Oil, Shea Butter (Cocoa Butter or Beeswax) and
Baking Soda

4 tablespoons Apricot Oil
2 tablespoons Shea Butter (or Cocoa Butter/Beeswax)
1 ¾ cups Water
1 teaspoon Baking Soda
4 tablespoons Castile Soap
½ cup Aloe Vera Gel (or Honey)
3 drops Essential Oil

In saucepan over low heat mix apricot oil and shea butter. Remove from heat. Pour into a bowl and let cool. In another saucepan, heat water. Add baking soda and castile soap. Stir until completely diluted. Add aloe vera gel. Pour soap mixture into the cooled apricote/shea butter mixture. Add essential oils. Make into cream. Pour in jar with lid. Keep in cool dry place.

WAXING

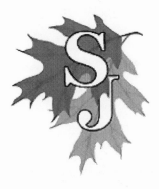

ରେ ରେ

Reusable Waxing Fabric Strips

Use washable fabrics . Thick varieties of cotton cloth work well as

Cut fabric into strips of 4 or 5 inches wide. Then sew a hem all around the edges of the fabric strips (this avoids unraveling with repeated washings of the strips)

Make numerous strips in various lengths for arms and legs. You may want to make some even smaller ones for eyebrows.

After using the strips for waxing, soak them in water to dissolve the wax, then wash.

ରେ ରେ

Sugar, Honey and Lemon Juice

1 cup granulated Sugar
1 cup Honey
½ cup Lemon Juice
Strips of fabric (cotton)
Cornstarch

Over medium-heat in a heaving saucepan heat sugar (don't stir) to caramelized. Stir in honey and lemon juice. Mix well. Remove from heat. Let wax cool slightly. Apply wax.

ଓଃ

NOTE: Sprinkle cornstarch to the area to remove moisture before applying wax.

ଓଃ

How to Wax

Work in small sections.

Apply the wax to the desired area.

Cover the wax with a strip of cloth.

Once cooled remove the strip by holding skin taught and pulling against the hair growth.

ଓଃ

Honey and Brown Sugar

1 teaspoon Brown Sugar
1 teaspoon Water
1 teaspoon Honey
1 cup of Water

In a saucepan heat water to simmering (less 1 teaspoon). Combine ingredients in a glass mug/jar and place in saucepan to melt. Remove from heat. Let cool slightly. Apply wax.

જા

Tip: use a tongue depressor, popsicle stick or small spatula to apply wax.

જા

Corn Syrup

2 oz Corn Cyrup
1 cup Water

Heat water to simmering. Place corn syrup in a glass jar/mug and sit down in water. Once hot remove from heat. Cool slightly. Apply syrup.

જા

❋ ❋ ❋

TOOTHPASTE
&
TOOTHPOWDERS

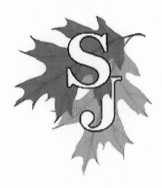

ભૂઈ ભૂઈ ભૂઈ ભૂઈ ભૂઈ ભૂઈ ભૂઈ ભૂઈ ભૂઈ ભૂઈ ભૂઈ ભૂઈ ભૂઈ ભૂઈ ભૂઈ ભૂઈ ભૂઈ ભૂઈ

Baking Soda, Cinnamon and Tea Tree Oil

1 teaspoon Baking Soda
¼ teaspoon Cinnamon
1 drop Tea Tree Oil

Mix baking soda, cinnamon, and tea tree oil.   Put in a jar/bottle.
Apply to toothbrush. Brush teeth

ભૂઈ ભૂઈ ભૂઈ ભૂઈ ભૂઈ ભૂઈ ભૂઈ ભૂઈ ભૂઈ ભૂઈ ભૂઈ ભૂઈ ભૂઈ ભૂઈ ભૂઈ ભૂઈ ભૂઈ ભૂઈ

Baking Soda, Sea Salt and Peppermint Extract

2/3 cup Baking Soda
1 teaspoon Fine Sea Salt
1 – 2 teaspoons peppermint extract (or an extract of your choice)
Water

Mix together baking soda, optional salt, and peppermint. Add a little
water at a time, stirring after each addition, until paste reaches desired
consistency. Apply to toothbrush. Brush teeth.

ભૂઈ ભૂઈ ભૂઈ ભૂઈ ભૂઈ ભૂઈ ભૂઈ ભૂઈ ભૂઈ ભૂઈ ભૂઈ ભૂઈ ભૂઈ ભૂઈ ભૂઈ ભૂઈ ભૂઈ ભૂઈ

> **Tip: the secret to a great smile starts with healthy gums**

ભૂઈ ભૂઈ ભૂઈ ભૂઈ ભૂઈ ભૂઈ ભૂઈ ભૂઈ ભૂઈ ભૂઈ ભૂઈ ભૂઈ ભૂઈ ભૂઈ ભૂઈ ભૂઈ ભૂઈ ભૂઈ

Calcium Powder, Baking Soda, Coconut Oil and Essential Oil

5 teaspoons Calcium Powder/Calcium Magnesium Powder

CR

2 teaspoons Baking Soda
3-5 teaspoons Coconut Oil
Essential Oil for flavor (mint, cinnamon, and orange)

Mix calcium, baking soda, coconut oil and essential oil. Put in jar with lid. Apply to toothbrush. Brush teeth

CRCRCRCRCRCRCRCRCRCRCRCRCRCRCRCRCRCRCRCRCRCRCRCR

The tooth is the only part of the human body that can't repair itself

CRCRCRCRCRCRCRCRCRCRCRCRCRCRCRCRCRCRCRCRCRCRCRCR

Vegetable Glycerin, Baking Soda, Guar Gum, and Essential Oil

2 teaspoons Vegetable Glycerin
4 tablespoon Baking Soda
½ teaspoon Guar Gum
8 tablespoons Water
5 drops Peppermint Oil(or clove, or citrus essential oil)
1 cup Water

Put ingredients(less essential oil) in saucepan and heat on low heat until mixture becomes a paste. Remove from heat and let cool. Add essential oil. Store in jar with lid. Apply to toothbrush. Brush teeth

CRCRCRCRCRCRCRCRCRCRCRCRCRCRCRCRCRCRCRCRCRCRCRCR

Baking Soda, Hydrogen Peroxide, Coconut Oil and Essential Oil

6 teaspoons Baking Soda

¼ teaspoon Hydrogen Peroxide
2 tablespoons Coconut Oil
10 drops Peppermint Oil (or Essential Oil of your choice)

Mix ingredients. Add essential oil to taste and store in a jar with lid. Apply to toothbrush. Brush teeth.

Tip: UV light breaks down hydrogen peroxide so keep toothpaste in dark cool place.

Baking Soda, Stevia Powder, Vegetable Glycerin and Essential Oil

6 teaspoons Baking Soda
1 teaspoon Stevia Powder
4 teaspoon Vegetable Glycerin (or 2 tablespoon Coconut Oil)
10 to 20 drops Peppermint Essential Oil

Mix ingredients and place in jar with lid. Apply to toothbrush. Brush teeth.

‱‱‱‱‱‱‱‱‱‱‱‱‱‱‱‱‱‱‱‱‱‱

TEETH WHITENERS

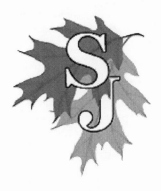

ɔʒ

PEARLY WHITE

I'm pretty obsessed about keeping myself groomed. Yes, to the point of keeping my pearly-whites – well, pearly white. I just love that just cleaned feeling of just brushed teeth don't you? Slick, shiny and sparkle-ly – okay I know you can't 'feel' shiny and sparkle-ly. Just sayin'.

Most times than not, a person will look at your mouth when you are talking or when first meeting. And what do they see? Yep, your teeth! I'm a smiler (one-who-smiles-a lot) and I get a little self-conscious that my teeth are not as white or clean as they could be (especially after eating that piece of blueberry pie the night before. Ugh!) So, while considering all my personal grooming aids for my survival kit, I knowing I may not have access to store-bought products, I began to wonder what alternatives I would have for tooth paste if the 'poo' should ever hit the fan. And, as with most of my journeys, I found there are tons of er ... lots of suggestions, thoughts and recipes for toothpaste/tooth powders. Some good and some, well not so feasible for a "poo-hits-the-fan" scenario.

I tried to focus the majority of my attention to looking for ingredients that we may have in our survival supplies already, or that we could add, if we don't.

From reviewing at all the ba-gillions of tid-bits of information out there, a pattern began to emerge - salt, baking soda and hydrogen peroxide (along with the proverbial drop or two of your favorite essential oil such as peppermint or spearmint.)

The method that surfaced over and over was, put a little baking soda and salt on your tooth brush and brush. Then gargling with a little hydrogen peroxide (making sure not to swallow any) and follow with dental floss. That's it. This is a method that has been passed down generation to generation. Pretty easy huh? With this info, we should be set to go with oral hygiene in a survival situation, right?

CR

But what about keeping your teeth white? The answer? Strawberries! Yepper, those yummy staples you grow out in your garden (and if you're not, you should be.) Strawberries contain malic acid which acts as an astringent to remove surface discoloration. If you use a little baking soda with strawberries it becomes a natural tooth-cleanser, buffing away stains. How cool is that? All you need to do is, take one ripe strawberry and crush it in to a pulp using a folk or back of a spoon in a bowl and then mix a ½ teaspoon of baking soda into the pulp and blend it together really well – like a paste. Do this manually opposed to using a blender keeping in mind, you may not have access to electricity in a poo-hits-the-fan scenario. Once your mixture is done, put some on your toothbrush and spread the mixture onto your teeth. Just like you would with your "whitening-type strips", leave this mixture on your teeth for a few minutes, and then brush thoroughly with your homemade toothpaste to remove the berry–baking soda mix and then rinse. Also, remember to floss after this treatment to get rid of the little seeds that may have gotten lodged between your teeth.

Now as with all good things, especially teeth whiteners, you must be careful not to use this whitening process too often, as the acid in the strawberries could damage the enamel on your teeth. NOT a good thing!! The common consensus is not to use this more than once a week.

How about "breath smell"? What do you do when you don't have a breath mint to pop in your mouth? The answer. Parsley. Parsley is great for bad breath. It's leaves are rich in chlorophyll and act as a powerful neutralizer of bad breath (and garlic-odor.) So keep this in mind as you're woofing down those garlic knots with your favorite pasta meal, and then realize you have a social engagement to go to afterwards. To ward off the garlic, ask the waiter to bring you a few sprigs of parsley to chew on after dinner. Oh, an added bonus, parsley when swallowed helps reduce intestinal gases (toot toot).

ଔଔଔଔଔଔଔଔଔଔଔଔଔଔଔଔଔଔଔଔଔଔଔଔଔଔଔଔ

Now, we may not be eating garlic knots in a survival situation, but we all wake up with 'dragon breath'. So, just like with the baking soda and salt remedy for brushing teeth, there is a simple remedy for mouthwash as well. Just boil some parsley and whole cloves together, let the mixture cool and then strain it to make a great gargle mouthwash for that "oh so fresh survivor breath".

Now, smile pretty!!!

CR

3% Hydrogen Peroxide

Use as a mouthwash. Swish around in mouth for 30 seconds. Spit out.

NOTE: 3% hydrogen peroxide is a natural bleaching agent.

CRCRCRCRCRCRCRCRCRCRCRCRCRCRCRCRCRCRCRCRCRCRCRCRCR

Baking Soda and Hydrogen Peroxide

1 tablespoon Baking Soda
2-3 tablespoon Hydrogen Peroxide

Add baking soda and hydrogen peroxide together to make a paste. Apply to toothbrush. Brush teeth.

CRCRCRCRCRCRCRCRCRCRCRCRCRCRCRCRCRCRCRCRCRCRCRCRCR

Sage Leaves

Wipe a fresh sage leaf over your teeth and gums. Or, dry and grind some sage leaves and make a tooth powder.

CRCRCRCRCRCRCRCRCRCRCRCRCRCRCRCRCRCRCRCRCRCRCRCRCR

Strawberries

Make a paste with a few strawberries. Apply the paste to your teeth and rub gently.

NOTE: Strawberries contain vitamin C which helps make your teeth whiter.

CR

Strawberries and Baking Soda

2-3 Strawberries
½ teaspoon Baking Soda

Mash strawberries. Add baking soda and mix well. Apply mixture to teeth. Leave on for few minutes. Rinse mouth and brush your teeth.

CRCRCRCRCRCRCRCRCRCRCRCRCRCRCRCRCRCRCRCRCRCRCRCRCR

Lemon

Lemon Juice
Salt

Combine a few drops of lemon juice and salt. Apply to teeth and rub the paste vigorously over your teeth and gums. Leave on 2 minutes. Rinse mouth.

CRCRCRCRCRCRCRCRCRCRCRCRCRCRCRCRCRCRCRCRCRCRCRCRCR

Orange Peel

Rub orange peel on your teeth every night before going to bed. With continued use your teeth will appear more shiny, stronger and whiter.

NOTE: The vitamin C and calcium present in orange peels help combat microorganisms in your mouth.

CRCRCRCRCRCRCRCRCRCRCRCRCRCRCRCRCRCRCRCRCRCRCRCRCR

> **Tip: don't have any charcoal - you can use the ashes of burnt bread**

ကြသြ

Charcoal

Take some charcoal powder and mix in with your regular toothpaste. Gently brush teeth. Along with charcoal you can also use the ashes of burnt bread and burnt rosemary in order to make your teeth whiter.

NOTE: Charcoal is one of the best known home remedies for yellow teeth.

ကြသြသြသြသြသြသြသြသြသြသြသြသြသြသြသြသြသြသြ

MOUTHWASH

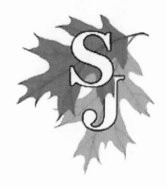

CR

Apple Cider Vinegar

1 tablespoon Apple Cider Vinegar

Gargle with a tablespoon of apple cider vinegar in the morning to loosen stains on teeth and refresh your mouth and gums.

CRCRCRCRCRCRCRCRCRCRCRCRCRCRCRCRCRCRCRCRCRCRCRCRCRCRCR

Vodka, Calendula Herbal Oil, Goldenseal Herbal Oil, Myrrh Herbal Oil and Peppermint Essential Oil

½ cup Water (distilled)
2 tablespoons Vodka
1 teaspoon Calendula Herbal Oil
1 teaspoon Goldenseal Herbal Oil
½ teaspoon Myrrh Herbal Oil
1 to 2 drops Peppermint Essential Oil

Combine all the ingredients. Place in a bottle. Use 3 tablespoons of the rinse in ½ ounce of water. Swish 30 seconds. Spit out. (…yes you have too)

CRCRCRCRCRCRCRCRCRCRCRCRCRCRCRCRCRCRCRCRCRCRCRCRCRCRCR

Aloe Vera Juice, Witch Hazel, Baking Soda and Essential Oil

½ cup Aloe Vera Juice
¼ cup Water (distilled)
½ tablespoon Witch Hazel
1 teaspoon Baking Soda
10 drops Peppermint Essential Oil

Mix ingredients together. Pour into a bottle with lid. Swish mixture in mouth 30 seconds. Spit out.

ℭℜ

Peppermint Essential Oil

½ cup Water (distilled)
3 drops of Peppermint Essential Oil

Mix water and essential oil. Pour in bottle and shake well. Swish mixture in mouth 30 seconds. Spit out.

ℭℜ

Baking Soda, Peppermint Essential Oil, Tea Tree Oil, Stevia, and Vodka

8 ounces Water (distilled)
1 teaspoon Baking Soda
4 drops Peppermint Essential Oil
4 drops Tea Tree Oil
5 drops Liquid Stevia (if desired)
1 teaspoon Vodka (if desired)

Combine all ingredients. Pour in bottle and Shake. Swish mixture in mouth 30 seconds. Spit out. (...yes you have too)

ℭℜ

Baking Soda and Peppermint Essential Oil

1 cup Water
1 teaspoon Baking Soda
3 drops Peppermint Essential Oil

Mix all ingredients in a glass jar and shake well. Swish mixture in mouth 30 seconds. Spit out.

Apple Cider Vinegar

1 cup Water
2 tablespoons Apple Cider Vinegar

Combine ingredients and store in a glass jar. Shake well prior to use. Swish mixture in mouth 30 seconds. Spit out.

Hydrogen Peroxide

1 part Hydrogen Peroxide
1 part Water

Mix peroxide with water. Swish mixture in mouth 30 seconds. Spit out.

Essential Oil and Water

1 cup Water
20 drops Cinnamon Essential Oil (or clove, wintergreen, tea tree)

Add cinnamon to water. Pour in bottle. Shake well. Swish mixture in mouth 30 seconds. Spit out.

DEODORANT

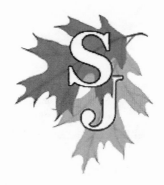

CR

Cornstarch and Essential Oil - Powder

½ cup Cornstarch
2-4 drops Essential Oil

In a jar mix cornstarch and essential oil. Place the lid on and shake well. Apply as needed.

CRCRCRCRCRCRCRCRCRCRCRCRCRCRCRCRCRCRCRCRCRCRCR

Baking Soda, Cornstarch, Coconut Oil
and Essential Oils - Cream

¼ cup Baking Soda
¼ cup Cornstarch (or Arrowroot Powder)
5 tablespoon Coconut Oil
2-3 drops of Tea Tree Oil (optional)

Mix ingredients well. Pour in small container with lid. Apply as needed.

CRCRCRCRCRCRCRCRCRCRCRCRCRCRCRCRCRCRCRCRCRCRCR

Coconut Oil, Baking Soda, Shea Butter, and
Arrowroot Powder - Cream

3 tablespoons Coconut Oil
3 tablespoons Baking Soda
2 tablespoons Shea Butter
2 tablespoons Arrowroot powder (optional)
2-3 drops Essential Oils (optional)

Mix ingredients well. Pour in small container with lid. Apply as needed.

CRCRCRCRCRCRCRCRCRCRCRCRCRCRCRCRCRCRCRCRCRCRCR

CR

Corn Starch and Baking Soda - Powder

3 tablespoon Corn starch
3 tablespoons Baking Soda

Combine equal amounts of corn starch and baking soda. Mix well and put in air tight container. Apply as needed.

CRCRCRCRCRCRCRCRCRCRCRCRCRCRCRCRCRCRCRCRCRCRCRCRCR

Tip: apply powdered deodorant using a powder puff

CRCRCRCRCRCRCRCRCRCRCRCRCRCRCRCRCRCRCRCRCRCRCRCRCR

Corn Starch, Baking Soda, Antibacterial Essential Oil, Antifungal Essential Oil, Vitamin E Oil, and Coconut Oil.

1/3 cup Corn Starch
1/3 cup Baking Soda
5 to 10 drops of Antibacterial Essential Oil (Tea Tree, Lavender, or Eucalyptus or a combo)
5 to 10 drops of Antifungal Essential Oil (Tea Tree, Peppermint, Sandalwood, or Eucalyptus or a combo)
1 - 2 tablespoons Vitamin E Oil (or Olive Oil)
3 tablespoons Coconut Oil

Mix all ingredients until smooth creamy. Put in air tight container. Apply as needed.

CRCRCRCRCRCRCRCRCRCRCRCRCRCRCRCRCRCRCRCRCRCRCRCRCR

Coconut Oil and Epsom Salt

½ cup Coconut Oil (liquefied)
2 tablespoons of Epsom Salt.

Mix ingredients until epsom salt dissolved. Put in air tight container. Apply as needed.

PERFUME

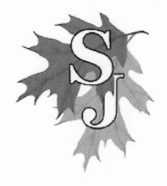

ප්‍ර

Almond Oil and Essential Oil

1 tablespoon Almond Oil
1 teaspoon Essential Oil

Mix almond oil and essential oil. Pour into spray bottle.

ප්‍ර

Vodka and Essential Oils

2 tablespoons 100 proof Vodka (or 80 proof but have to shake bottle each time)
Essential oils
Glass spray bottle

Mix vodka and essential oils. Pour into spray bottle.

ප්‍ර

FEMININE CARE

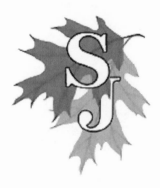

ᏣᎧᏣᎧᏣᎧᏣᎧᏣᎧᏣᎧᏣᎧᏣᎧᏣᎧᏣᎧᏣᎧᏣᎧᏣᎧᏣᎧᏣᎧᏣᎧ

THE HINEY HYDRANT

I've stopped using toilet paper. Honest. And I may never use it again … well at home at least. I was determined that I was not going to wait unit the "poo-to-hit-the-fan" or any place else for that matter before securing an alternative to toilet paper.

To me, it just doesn't make sense to stockpiling toilet paper ceiling to floor for your preps. It's not like food where you can replenish it from a garden. When it's gone – it's gone. End of story.

As we all know, or should know, one of the many prepper mantras has always been - have backups for your backups. No exception. So it only seemed to reason I would want to have backups for my backend as well. I am a huge believer in cleanliness. Call me vain, call me a girlie-girl, just don't call me to say you're out of toilet paper. Sorry.

I began searching high and low for toilet paper alternatives. And there are a lot of things out there. I was amazed at what people are willing to use!

Let's start with some bushcraft-type methods or outdoorsy methods. There are leaves. Large, relatively green leaves from plants such as abutilon, hollyhocks, mullein, comfrey, wild grape and mulberry (which to tell you the truth I wouldn't know one from the other) said to make a good alternatives to toilet paper. But to me, it seemed more spreading than cleaning (sorry for the mental image). Not good. Also, you need to make sure to avoid the scratchy or prickly varieties or you'll have more issues than just "poo-pants".

Then, there is snow. In the winter time snow can be used (brrrr, I know.) Make a small snowball about the size of the palm of your hand and form an oval shape. Then, well … nuff said you know the rest.

CR

Moving inside the home, there are the moist wipes ... but to me this is the same as toilet paper, it takes up a lot of valuable space and they too will run out. So moving on ...

There's the cloth or rag method ... or what I consider to be the big brother to 'baby-poopy diapers'. You cut up wash cloths, old t-shirts or blankets into small squares to use. Once used, cling-ons and all, are put into a pail of chlorinated water to be dealt with later.

You can also use newspaper or phone books ... but if you think we have a bad rap being called "horders" with our food stores and prepping supplies, just wait 'til someone catches a glimpse of your stacks of newspapers and phone books! As a caveat, I will say in paper's defense, if there is ever a devaluation of the dollar we could always just use crumpled up paper money – I'm sure there will be plenty to go around. Just sayin.

Next, portable bidets. These are plastic bottles with a hook shape nozzle filled with about a cup of water that you squeeze to produce a stream of water to cleanse yourself. The problem I've read with most of these portable bidets is there's no pressure (the key to a good cleansing is pressure) and one cup of water does not go far in cleansing either. It would be kinda like holding up a Kleenex in a hurricane to keep from getting wet. It just doesn't do the job.

And then there's ... the left hand method where you wipe your fanny with your left hand ... no paper, just your hand. And that my friend, to me is the mac-daddy of grossness! It reminds me of going to the zoo. There was always that one monkey that seemed to entertain young and old alike. You know the one - "Whoo Flung Poo"?

So, with all this said, what marvelous method did I come up with? Well I didn't invented the devise ... but I did modify it for an entirely different purpose. The reveal (drum roll please) - a simple one (1) gallon garden sprayer I purchased for $9!

Wait....wait, before saying anything - hear me out. I cut 4.5 – 5 inches off the spray wand to shorten it. Then I placed the wand (the part that eventually connects to the tank) in boiling water to soften it to make a "curve" (this shape makes it gender friendly for those hard to reach areas due to physical obstacles hanging down.) And, whaa-laa a bidet with a control tip for a light summer misting all the way up to a full-on power blaster (men seem to prefer this setting – just sayin'.)

But what about the wetness? Well I purchased 18 white washcloths for $4. I placed them in a tall Tupperware container (a celery holder actually) and folded them into each other like Kleenex. I found a little trash can with a plastic bucket liner in it and filled the bucket 3/4 full with water and added some homemade oxyclean (2 parts water, 1 part hydrogen peroxide, 1 part washing soda). When I use a cloth – with very little or next to nothing on it from my business - I put it in the bucket. Then when I do laundry … I empty the cloths and liquid into the washing machine add a little detergent and some vinegar and they come out white as snow! Note: you don't have to do the wash cloths and bucket thing. I just like to keep things as sanitary as possible. Oh, and I spray the nozzle with a disinfectant after each use - just because.

A gallon of water can actually last a week depending on how many are using the "hh". And the container sans the water is so light you can attach it to your emergency go-bag and take with you in an emergency. Then, all you have to do it empty a bottle of water into the sprayer – pump it up and you're good to 'go' (giggle). How easy is that!? Just sayin'.

CR

> The word "tampon" is a derivative of the French word tapon which means a plug or stopper.

CRCRCRCRCRCRCRCRCRCRCRCRCRCRCRCRCRCRCRCRCRCRCR

Reusable Tampons

Reusable Tampon are alternatives to disposable tampons. They are washable and can be handmade by using fabric and filling them with absorbent material, or knitting or crocheting them, then adding a string for removal.

NOTE: Some have used such items as cotton baby socks rolled up as tampons.

CRCRCRCRCRCRCRCRCRCRCRCRCRCRCRCRCRCRCRCRCRCRCR

> **Tip: use all-cotton fabrics when making reusable tampons. Cotton fibers do not breed bacteria like rayon fibers do.**

CRCRCRCRCRCRCRCRCRCRCRCRCRCRCRCRCRCRCRCRCRCRCR

Tip: the tampon is regulated in the US by the Food & Drug Administration as a Class II Medical Device

Reusable Menstrual Cloth Pads

Menstrual cloth pads are reusable alternatives to disposable sanitary napkins. They are usually made from fabrics such as cotton or hemp and come in a range of options and styles.

NOTE: Menstrual cloth pad can be made, purchased or even created by using something as simple as a folded wash cloth.

NOTE: Once the cloth pads are worn and soiled, just rinse in cold water, then wash, dry and reuse.

Tip: a woman will use 16,800 pads or tampons in her lifetime.

The tampon has long been held as a valuable survival item by using the tampon, its plastic outer sheath and/or the wrapper in creative uses such as:

Tampon:
Plugging a Wound
Medical Bandage
Emergency Water Filter
Survival Straw
Fire tender
Wick
Cordage
Nose Bleeds
Ear Plugs
Cotton Pad
Eye Compress

Plastic Sheath:
Fishing Bobber
Blow Tube for Fire Starting

Plastic Wrapper:
Carry Water Proof Tinder and Matches
Fishing Bobber

CR

> ## Menstrual cloth pads are what most of the world uses

CRCRCRCRCRCRCRCRCRCRCRCRCRCRCRCRCRCRCRCRCRCRCRCRCR

Reusable Menstrual Cup

A Menstrual Cup, is a pliable cup made of rubber or silicone that is inserted into the vagina forming a suction that holds it in place. Most have a bottom portion used to grasp and remove it. Once removed you rinse or wipe it out and reinsert.

CRCRCRCRCRCRCRCRCRCRCRCRCRCRCRCRCRCRCRCRCRCRCRCRCR

> ## A Menstrual Cup usually holds one fluid ounce, often compared to a super-plus tampon

CRCRCRCRCRCRCRCRCRCRCRCRCRCRCRCRCRCRCRCRCRCRCRCRCR

Sea Sponges

Reusable sea sponges are an alternative to tampons. You dampen the sponge with water, squeeze out the water or you can use it dry. Insert the sponge (wet or dry) into the vagina to absorb the menstrual flow.

NOTE: Periodically, the sponge should be removed, squeezed out, rinsed out with water and reinserted.

CRCRCRCRCRCRCRCRCRCRCRCRCRCRCRCRCRCRCRCRCRCRCRCRCR

215

 ca

NOTE: To disinfect the sponge some use ingredients such as tea tree oil, vinegar or hydrogen peroxide.

cacacacacacacacacacacacacacacacacaca

Tip: wash your hands before inserting any vaginal menstrual option

cacacacacacaccacacacacacacacacacacacaca

❋ ❋ ❋

ℭℜℭℜℭℜℭℜℭℜℭℜℭℜℭℜℭℜℭℜℭℜℭℜℭℜℭℜℭℜℭℜℭℜℭℜ

INGROWN
&
EMBEDDED HAIRS

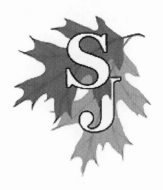

ᗰᗰᗰᗰᗰᗰᗰᗰᗰᗰᗰᗰᗰᗰᗰᗰᗰᗰᗰᗰᗰᗰᗰᗰᗰᗰᗰᗰ

Removal of Ingrown Hair

Apply a warm compress to the area of the ingrown hair to soften the area and to allow the hair to come to the surface.

Needle or tweezers - Begin by sterilizing the instrument by first washing your hands. Then, holding the instrument firming in one hand with the other hand use a lighter to burn the tip of the instrument that will be piercing the skin. Next, as an additional measure, soak the instrument in rubbing alcohol or hydrogen peroxide for a few minutes.

Gently coax the hair out.

Follow with a topical antibiotic ointment.

ᗰᗰᗰᗰᗰᗰᗰᗰᗰᗰᗰᗰᗰᗰᗰᗰᗰᗰᗰᗰᗰᗰᗰᗰᗰᗰᗰᗰ

Tylenol

2-3 Tylenol Tablets (or any non-coated Acetaminophen or Paracetamol tablet)

CRRCRRCRRCRRCRRCRRCRRCRRCRRCRRCRRCRRCRRCRRCRRCRRCRRCRRCRR

Crush the tablets. Add water to make a paste. Rub paste over the in-grown hair area in a circular motion for about 1-2 minutes. Rinse and patting dry.

CRRCRRCRRCRRCRRCRRCRRCRRCRRCRRCRRCRRCRRCRRCRRCRRCRRCRRCRR

> **Tip: to 'help' remove an in-grown hair start by exfoliating the area around the ingrown hair to remove any dead skin cells, dirt, and oils.**

CRRCRRCRRCRRCRRCRRCRRCRRCRRCRRCRRCRRCRRCRRCRRCRRCRRCRRCRR

Salt

½ teaspoons Salt
Liquid Soap

Make a paste with salt and liquid soap. Rub paste over the in-grown hair area in a circular motion for about 1-2 minutes. Rinse and patting dry.

CRRCRRCRRCRRCRRCRRCRRCRRCRRCRRCRRCRRCRRCRRCRRCRRCRRCRRCRR

> When a hair penetrates your skin, your skin reacts as it would to a foreign body and becomes inflamed.

CR

Olive oil and Sugar

Olive oil
Sugar (either white or brown sugar)

Wet area around the in-grown hair with warm water. Mix a small amount of olive oil and sugar together. Gently apply to the area and rub in a circular motion for about 20 or 30 seconds. Rinse the area and patting dry.

CRCRCRCRCRCRCRCRCRCRCRCRCRCRCRCRCRCRCRCRCRCRCRCR

Toothpaste

Apply a small amount of toothpaste to the in-grown hair area to help reduce swelling allowing the hair to surface.

CRCRCRCRCRCRCRCRCRCRCRCRCRCRCRCRCRCRCRCRCRCRCRCR

Warm Compress

Wet cloth/compress with hot water. Apply to the in-grown hair for 1-2 minutes to soften the skin and bring the hair closer to the surface.

CRCRCRCRCRCRCRCRCRCRCRCRCRCRCRCRCRCRCRCRCRCRCRCR

☙ 9 ❧
MAKE-UP

Cosmetics are as old as vanity. Vanity is as old as mankind.

MAKE-UP REMOVERS

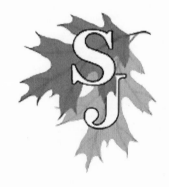

CR

Olive Oil, Canola Oil and Castor oil

1 tablespoon Olive Oil
1 tablespoon Canola Oil
1 tablespoon Castor Oil

Mix oils together. Place in an airtight container. Apply mixture cotton ball and wipe over the eyelids and the upper and lower eyelashes to remove eye make up.

CRCRCRCRCRCRCRCRCRCRCRCRCRCRCRCRCRCRCRCRCRCRCRCRCR

Extra Virgin Olive Oil

Extra virgin olive oil (or almond oil)

Add a few drops of olive oil to a cotton pad or cotton ball. Wipe your face in a circular motion.

NOTE: To remove eye makeup, place the cotton pad against your closed eye for 10 seconds and gently wipe.

CRCRCRCRCRCRCRCRCRCRCRCRCRCRCRCRCRCRCRCRCRCRCRCRCR

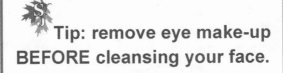

Tip: remove eye make-up BEFORE cleansing your face.

CRCRCRCRCRCRCRCRCRCRCRCRCRCRCRCRCRCRCRCRCRCRCRCRCR

Milk & Almond Oil

1 tablespoon Milk
2 - 3 drops of Sweet Almond Oil

Mix milk and sweet almond oil. Apply mixture on cotton ball. Remove makeup. Rinse face.

> **Tip: oil is excellent for removing make-up and nourishing all types of skin.**

Yogurt

Plain unflavored yogurt

Dip a cotton ball in the yogurt. Gently wipe face. Rinse.

Witch Hazel and Carrier Oil

¼ cup Witch Hazel
¼ cup Carrier Oil (your choice)

Mix witch hazel and carrier oil. Place in a container with lid. Apply to face with cotton ball.

Witch Hazel, Carrier Oil and Water

2 tablespoons Witch Hazel
2 tablespoons Carrier Oil (your choice)
2 tablespoons Water

ଊଊଊଊଊଊଊଊଊଊଊଊଊଊଊଊଊଊଊଊଊଊଊଊଊଊଊ

Mix witch hazel, carrier oil and water. Pour into container. Apply to face with cotton ball.

ଊଊଊଊଊଊଊଊଊଊଊଊଊଊଊଊଊଊଊଊଊଊଊଊଊଊଊ

MAKE-UP
REMOVER WIPES

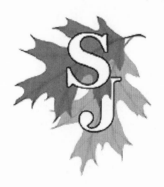

ଔଔଔଔଔଔଔଔଔଔଔଔଔଔଔଔଔଔଔଔଔଔଔଔଔଔଔଔ

Coconut Oil and Tea Tree Oil

4 cups Warm Water
1-2 tablespoons Coconut Oil.
1-2 squirts of baby wash or face wash (optional)
½ Roll of Paper Towels or Napkins
Container with lid

Cut roll of paper towels in half. Place one half in a plastic container or bottle (large enough to fit). Mix water, oil, and tea tree oil together. Pour over paper towels in container. Let sit for 10 minutes. Remove the cardboard core. Put lid on container. Turn container upside down and continue soaking for 30 minutes.

NOTE: You can cut and "X" into the top of the lid and pull a wipe through the "X" from the center of the roll.

ଔଔଔଔଔଔଔଔଔଔଔଔଔଔଔଔଔଔଔଔଔଔଔଔଔଔଔଔ

Castile Soap, Aloe Vera Gel, Witch Hazel Extract, and Sweet Almond Oil

1 ½ cups Water (boiled and cooled)
1 tablespoon Castile Soap
1 tablespoon Aloe Vera Gel
1 tablespoon Witch Hazel Extract
1 tablespoon Sweet Almond Oil (or olive oil)
1 Roll Paper Towels (or Napkins or Round Cotton Pads)

Cut roll of paper towels in half. Place one half in a plastic container or bottle (large enough to fit). Mix water, oil, and tea tree oil together. Pour over paper towels in container. Let sit for 10 minutes. Remove the cardboard core. Put lid on container. Turn container upside down and continue soaking for 30 minutes.

LIP BALM
&
LIP GLOSS

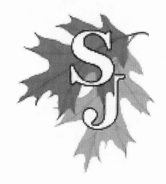

Beeswax, Cocoa Butter, and Coconut Oil

1 teaspoon Beewax
1 teaspoon Cocoa Butter (or Shea Butter)
1 teaspoon Coconut Oil
1 cup Water

In a saucepan bring water to a low simmer. Put beeswax, cocoa butter and coconut oil in a glass jar/mug and set it down in water until melted. Remove from heat. Pour into used lipstick, chap stick container or makeup pot. Let cool 30 minutes. Store in a cool place.

Beeswax, Shea Butter, Carrier Oil and Essential Oil

1 teaspoon Beeswax
2 teaspoon Shea Butter
1 teaspoon Carrier Oil
1/8 teaspoon Essential Oil
1 cup Water

In a saucepan on low heat, melt beeswax, shea butter and carrier oil. Remove from heat. Cool 2-3 minutes. Add Essential oil. Pour into lipstick or chapstick tube or pot with lid.

Beeswax, Carrier Oil and Essential Oil

1 teaspoon Beeswax or Beeswax Beads
3 teaspoons Carrier Oil
1/8 teaspoon Essential Oil

In saucepan on low heat, melt beeswax and carrier oil. Remove from heat. Cool 2-3 minutes. Add essential oil and mix well. Pour into lipstick/chapstick tubes or pots with lids.

Beeswax, Coconut Oil, Vitamin E Oil and Vanilla Extract

1 tablespoon Beeswax
1 tablespoon Coconut Oil
1/8 teaspoon Vitamin E Oil
1/8 teaspoon Vanilla Extract

In saucepan on low heat, melt beeswax, coconut oil and vitamin E oil. Stir in the vanilla extract and mix well. Pour into lipstick/chapstick tubes or pots with lids.

Beeswax, Carrier Oil, Essential Oil and Honey

3 tablespoons Beeswax
5 teaspoons Carrier Oil
6-7 drops Essential Oil
1 teaspoon honey

In saucepan on low heat, melt beeswax and carrier oil. Remove from heat. Add honey and essential oil. Pour into lipstick/chapstick tubes or pots with lids.

COLORED - LIPSTICK
&
LIP GLOSS

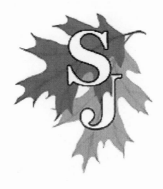

ରେଉଉଉଉଉଉଉଉଉଉଉଉଉଉଉଉଉଉଉଉଉଉଉଉଉଉ

Beet Juice, Beeswax, Caster Oil, Sesame Oil

¼ cup Beewax
¼ cup Castor Oil
2 tablespoons Sesame Oil
Beet Juice
1 cup Water

In saucepan heat water to a low simmer. Put beeswax in a glass mug/jar and set down in water. When melted remove from heat. Add oils and add beet juice to desired color. Pour into lipstick/chapstick tubes or pots with lids. Let cool 30 minutes. Keep in cool place.

ରେଉଉଉଉଉଉଉଉଉଉଉଉଉଉଉଉଉଉଉଉଉଉଉଉଉଉ

Beeswax, Cocoa Butter, and Coconut Oil

1 teaspoon Beewax
1 teaspoon Cocoa Butter (or Shea Butter)
1 teaspoon Coconut Oil
1 drop Essential Oil (optional)
1 cup Water

Colors

Red : 1/8 teaspoon beet root powder or 1 drop of natural red food coloring.

Brown or Tan: ¼ teaspoon cocoa powder . For variations add small amount of cinnamon or turmeric.

In a saucepan heat water to low simmer. Put beeswax, cocoa butter and coconut oil in a glass jar/mug and set down in water. When melted remove from heat. Add color and essential oil (optional). Pour into used lipstick or chap stick container or used lip gloss pot with lid. Let cool 30 minutes. Store in a cool place.

ෆ෫

Beeswax, Shea Butter, Carrier Oil and Essential Oil

1 teaspoon Beeswax
2 teaspoon Shea Butter
1 teaspoon Carrier Oil
1/8 teaspoon Essential Oil
1 cup Water

Colors

Red - 1/8 teaspoon of beet root powder

Brown or Tan – ¼ teaspoon Cocoa powder (and small amount of cinnamon or turmeric)

In saucepan heat water to a low simmer. In a glass mug/jar put beeswax, shea butter and carrier oil. Set jar down in water. When melted remove from heat. Cool 2-3 minutes. Add essential oil and color. Pour into lipstick/chapstick tubes or pots with lids. Store in cool place.

ෆ෫

Beeswax, Shea Butter, Almond Oil, Beet Root Powder, Cinnamon, Turmeric, and Cocoa Powder

1 teaspoon Beeswax
1 teaspoon Shea Butter
1 teaspoon Almond Oil (or Extra Virgin Olive Oil, Jojoba Oil)
1 cup Water

Colors

Bright Red - Beet Root Powder

Reddish Brown - Cinnamon

CRICRICRICRICRICRICRICRICRICRICRICRICRICRICRICRICRICRICRICR

Copper -Turmeric

Deep Brown - Cocoa Powder

Heat water in a saucepan to a low simmer. In a glass mug/jar add beeswax, shea butter and almond oil. Set in water. When melted remove from heat. Add color. Pour into used lipstick or chap stick container or used lip gloss pot. Let cool 30 minutes. Store in a cool place.

CRICRICRICRICRICRICRICRICRICRICRICRICRICRICRICRICRICRICRICR

Petroleum Jelly, Kool-Aid Mix, Vanilla Extract and Aloe Vera Gel

1 teaspoon Petroleum Jelly
Kool-Aid Powder Mix (Cherry, Raspberry Grape etc.)
Vanilla Extract (optional)
Aloe Vera Gel (optional)

Mix petroleum jelly, kool-aid powder, vanilla extract and aloe vera gel. Put in lip gloss pot. Keep in cool place.

CRICRICRICRICRICRICRICRICRICRICRICRICRICRICRICRICRICRICRICR

Beeswax, Carrier Oil, Essential Oil, Beet Root Powder, Cinnamon, and Turmeric

1 teaspoon Beeswax
3 teaspoons Carrier Oil
1/8 teaspoon Essential Oil

Colors

Red - 1/8 teaspoon of beet root powder
Brown or Tan — ¼ teaspoon cocoa powder. Add small amount of cinnamon or turmeric for variations.

CR CR CR CR CR CR CR CR CR CR CR CR CR CR CR CR CR CR CR CR CR CR CR CR

In saucepan heat water to a low simmer. Put beeswax and carrier oil in a glass jar/mug and set down in water. When melted remove from heat. Cool 2-3 minutes. Add essential oil and color and mix well. Pour into lipstick/chapstick tubes or pots.

CR CR CR CR CR CR CR CR CR CR CR CR CR CR CR CR CR CR CR CR CR CR CR CR

Almond Oil, Cranberries, Honey and Petroleum Jelly

1 tablespoon Almond Oil
10 fresh Cranberries
1 teaspoon Honey
1 teaspoon Petroleum Jelly (optional - for more shine)
1 cup Water

In a saucepan bring water to a low simmer. Add ingredients to a glass mug/jar. Put down in water. Heat until mixture begins to boil. Remove from heat. Stir well. Gently mash berries. Let mixture stand for 5 minutes. Strain mixture through a sieve. Stir and allow to cool completely. When cool, put in lip gloss pot. Keep in cool place.

CR CR CR CR CR CR CR CR CR CR CR CR CR CR CR CR CR CR CR CR CR CR CR CR

Beetroot Powder, Vegetable Glycerin and Vitamin E Oil

1 teaspoon Beetroot Powder
1 teaspoon Vegetable Glycerin
½ teaspoon Vitamin E oil

Combine vegetable glycerin and beetroot powder. Stir until smooth. Add the vitamin E oil. Store in small jar/container. Keep in cool place.

CR CR CR CR CR CR CR CR CR CR CR CR CR CR CR CR CR CR CR CR CR CR CR CR CR CR

Blackberries, Raspberry, Pomegranate Seeds and Olive Oil

3 Blackberries
1 Raspberry
3 Pomegranate Juice
½ teaspoon Extra Virgin Olive Oil

Mash the blackberries and raspberry in the bowl. Extract juice from pomegranate seeds and add to mixture. Stir in the olive oil. Put into jar or bottle. Store in cool place.

CR CR CR CR CR CR CR CR CR CR CR CR CR CR CR CR CR CR CR CR CR CR CR CR CR CR

FOUNDATION POWDER & CREAM

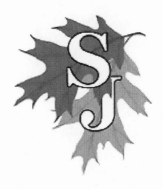

CR

Arrowroot Powder, Cocoa Powder, Cinnamon, Ginger, and Wheat Grass Powder

1 tablespoon Arrowroot Powder (or Corn Starch)
Any or all of the following:

Cocoa powder (darkens and adds richness)
Cinnamon (darkens and adds richness)
Ginger (for yellow pigments in skin)
Wheat grass Powder (for more red pigments in the skin)

Depending on the color of your skin, add cornstarch and cocoa powder, cinnamon, ginger or wheat grass powder in small increments. Place in a jar with airtight lid.

NOTE: To match your skin tone put a small amount of powder on the back of your hand.

CRCRCRCRCRCRCRCRCRCRCRCRCRCRCRCRCRCRCRCRCRCRCRCR

Arrowroot Powder, Cocoa Powder, Cinnamon and Nutmeg

1 teaspoon Arrowroot Powder (or Cornstarch) for dark skin
1 tablespoon Arrowroot Powder (or Cornstarch) for light skin
Cocoa powder
Cinnamon
Nutmeg

Start with a base of arrowroot powder (or cornstarch). Add small amount of cocoa powder, cinnamon, or nutmeg or any combination to match your skin tone. Place in a jar with airtight lid.

CRCRCRCRCRCRCRCRCRCRCRCRCRCRCRCRCRCRCRCRCRCRCRCR

CR

Arrow Root Powder, Cocoa Powder, Cinnamon, Nutmeg and Olive Oil

1 teaspoon Arrowroot Powder (or Cornstarch) (for Dark Skin
1 tablespoon Arrowroot Powder (or Cornstarch) for Light Skin
Cocoa powder
Cinnamon
Nutmeg
Olive Oil (or Jojoba Oil, Sweet Almond Oil)

Start with a base of arrowroot powder (or corn starch) Add small amount of cocoa powder, cinnamon, or nutmeg or any combination to match your skin tone. Add one or two drops of olive oil. Place in a jar with airtight lid.

CRCRCRCRCRCRCRCRCRCRCRCRCRCRCRCRCRCRCRCRCRCRCR

BLUSH
POWDER & CREAM

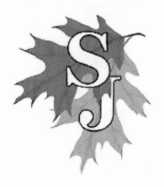

CR

Arrowroot Powder, Beet Root Powder, Cocoa Powder, and Cinnamon

1 tablespoon Arrowroot Powder (or Corn Starch)
2 tablespoon Beet Root Powder (or more depending on depth)
Cocoa Powder (for darker color)
Cinnamon (for darker color)

Mix arrowroot powder and beet root powder. Add cocoa powder and/or cinnamon for darker color. Place in a jar with airtight lid.

CRCRCRCRCRCRCRCRCRCRCRCRCRCRCRCRCRCRCRCRCRCRCRCRCR

Beet Powder, Arrowroot Powder, Ground Nutmeg, Ground Ginger, and Essential Oil

2 tablespoons Beet Powder
1 tablespoon Arrowroot Powder (or Corn Starch)
Ground Nutmeg (optional for shimmer for darker blush)
Ground Ginger (optional for shimmer for lighter blush)
3-5 drops Essential Oil

Mix beet powder to arrowroot powder. Depending on how dark or light you want the blush, add as much beet powder to achieve the right color. If you want a shimmer add a little nutmeg and/or ginger Mix well. Add in the essential oil. Store in jar/container with lid.

NOTE: we all have different skin tones so adjust portions to your particular needs.

CRCRCRCRCRCRCRCRCRCRCRCRCRCRCRCRCRCRCRCRCRCRCRCRCR

Powdered Bronzer

1 tablespoon Cinnamon Powder
1 teaspoon Cocoa Powder
1 teaspoon Nutmeg Powder

ⅭⅭⅭⅭⅭⅭⅭⅭⅭⅭⅭⅭⅭⅭⅭⅭⅭⅭⅭⅭⅭⅭⅭⅭⅭⅭⅭⅭⅭⅭⅭⅭ

2 teaspoons Cornstarch
15 drops Essential Oil

Mix all ingredients well. Use a flour sifter for a fine powder. Put in small jar or pot with lid. Use a blush brush to apply bronzer.

NOTE: Cinnamon adds glow, Cocoa adds depth/darkness, nutmeg adds a light touch

ⅭⅭⅭⅭⅭⅭⅭⅭⅭⅭⅭⅭⅭⅭⅭⅭⅭⅭⅭⅭⅭⅭⅭⅭⅭⅭⅭⅭⅭⅭ

MASCARA

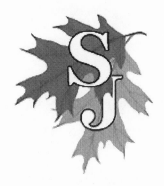

CR

Coconut Oil, Aloe Vera Gel, Beeswax, Activated Charcoal or Cocoa Powder

2 teaspoons Coconut Oil
4 teaspoons Aloe Vera Gel
¾ - 1 teaspoon Beeswax
¼ teaspoon – ½ teaspoon Activated Charcoal or Cocoa Powder
1 cup Water

In saucepan heat water to a low simmer. Put coconut oil, aloe vera gel and beeswax in a glass jar/mug. Heat until melted. Add activated charcoal or cocoa powder and mix completely. Remove from heat. Cool slightly and put in jar with airtight lid.

NOTE: Pour contents into a sandwich bag and snip the corner to put it in a clean used mascara tube.

CRCRCRCRCRCRCRCRCRCRCRCRCRCRCRCRCRCRCRCRCRCRCRCRCR

In 1917 American company Maybelline created the first mascara consisting of black coal and Vaseline

CRCRCRCRCRCRCRCRCRCRCRCRCRCRCRCRCRCRCRCRCRCRCRCRCR

Activated Charcoal, Cornstarch, and Coconut Oil

4 Activated Charcoal Capsules
¼ teaspoon Cornstarch
½ teaspoon Water
3-4 drops Coconut Oil (or Argon Oil, Jojoba Oil or Vigin Olive Oil)

CR

Mix charcoal and cornstarch together. Add oil and mix. Then add water. Store in jar/container with lid or a clean, used mascara tube.

CRCRCRCRCRCRCRCRCRCRCRCRCRCRCRCRCRCRCRCRCRCRCRCR

Activated Charcoal, Cornstarch, Coconut Oil and Beeswax

4 Activated Charcoal Capsules
¼ teaspoon Cornstarch
½ teaspoon Water
3-4 drops Coconut Oil
¼ teaspoon Beeswax
½ teaspoon Coconut Oil
1 cup water

Mix charcoal and cornstarch together. Add in oil and water. In a saucepan heat water to a low simmer. In a glass mug/jar add beeswax and coconut oil and sit down in water. When melted add to charcoal mixture. Store in jar/container with lid.

CRCRCRCRCRCRCRCRCRCRCRCRCRCRCRCRCRCRCRCRCRCRCRCR

EYELINER

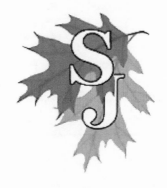

CR

Coconut Oil, Aloe Vera Gel, Activated Charcoal or Cocoa Powder

2 teaspoons Coconut Oil
4 teaspoons Aloe Vera Gel
1 – 2 capsules of Activated Charcoal (for black)
½ teaspoon Cocoa Powder (for Brown)

Mix coconut oil and aloe vera gel. Then add activated charcoal (for black) or cocoa powder (for brown). Pour in airtight container. Keep in cool place.

CRCRCRCRCRCRCRCRCRCRCRCRCRCRCRCRCRCRCRCRCRCRCRCR

Activated Charcoal and Coconut Oil

1-3 Activated Charcoal Capsules
¼ - ½ teaspoon Coconut Oil (depending on thickness)

Put charcoal in a jar with a lid. Add coconut oil. Stir into a liquid. Store in cool place.

NOTE: For blacker liner add more charcoal

CRCRCRCRCRCRCRCRCRCRCRCRCRCRCRCRCRCRCRCRCRCRCRCR

Pecan and Olive Oil

1 Pecan (almond or walnut)
Olive Oil

Using a pair of tongs hold a nut (of your choice) and using a candle lighter burn the nut to a crisp. Place the nut in a bowl. Crush the nut into a powder. Place in a jar with airtight lid. Add a few drops of olive oil and mix into a cream.

EYE SHADOW

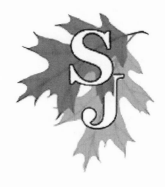

CR

Primer

½ teaspoon Chapstick (plain)
1 teaspoon Cornstarch
1 ½ teaspoon Liquid Foundation
1 cup Water

In a saucepan heat water to a low simmer. Remove from heat. Place a tube of chapstick in a glass mug/jar and put it in the water to soften. Once soften, add chapstick, cornstarch and foundation. Mix well. Place in jar with lid.

CRCRCRCRCRCRCRCRCRCRCRCRCRCRCRCRCRCRCRCRCRCRCRCRCR

Cocoa Powder and Cornstarch

(Brown Powder Eye Shadow)

Cocoa Powder
Cornstarch

Combine cocoa powder and cornstarch. Put into a small jar with lid.

CRCRCRCRCRCRCRCRCRCRCRCRCRCRCRCRCRCRCRCRCRCRCRCRCR

Spirulina and Cornstarch

(Green Powder Eye Shadow)

Spirulina (a natural dietary supplement)
Cornstarch (or arrowroot)

Combine spirulina and cornstarch. Put into a jar with lid.

CRCRCRCRCRCRCRCRCRCRCRCRCRCRCRCRCRCRCRCRCRCRCRCRCR

CR

Activated Charcoal and Arrowroot Powder

(Black/Grey Powdered Eye Shadow)

Activated Charcoal
Arrowroot Powder

Mix charcoal and arrowroot powder.

NOTE: Add more or less charcoal for desired shade

CRCRCRCRCRCRCRCRCRCRCRCRCRCRCRCRCRCRCRCRCRCR

Saffron and Beetroot Juice

(Gold/Orange Cream Eye Shadow)

Saffron
Beetroot Juice

Mix saffron and beetroot juice into a paste. Place in jar with lid.

CRCRCRCRCRCRCRCRCRCRCRCRCRCRCRCRCRCRCRCRCRCR

❧ 10 ❦
HAIR
STYLING & CUTTING

The hair is the

richest ornament of

women.

~ Martin Luther

TRIMMING

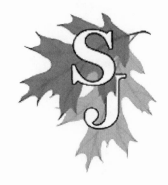

CR CR CR CR CR CR CR CR CR CR CR CR CR CR CR CR CR CR CR CR CR CR CR CR CR CR CR

Trim Dead Ends or Overall Length

Part your hair from the front of your head back to the nap of your neck. Then from the top of your head down to the top of the ear on each side - making four sections. Using an elastic band secure each section into a pony tail (one on each side of your head and two in the back). Make sure each section is the same level all the way around your head.

Holding one of the ponytail straight out from your head, slide the elastic band out towards the end of the ponytail. Cut the desired amount off. Then move to the next ponytail and once again moving the elastic band down cut the same amount off. Continue this process until all ponytails are trimmed.

CR CR CR CR CR CR CR CR CR CR CR CR CR CR CR CR CR CR CR CR CR CR CR CR CR CR CR

Trim Bangs I

Comb bangs straight out in front of you. Twist them once or twice to the right. With your scissors pointing up, cut into the hairs vertically. The twist the hair the other direction (left) and again cut any strangler hairs vertically.

CR CR CR CR CR CR CR CR CR CR CR CR CR CR CR CR CR CR CR CR CR CR CR CR CR CR CR

Trim Bangs II

Part your hair in the middle from front to back. Take an equal amount of hair from each side of the part and comb it forward. Smooth the hair between your index and middle fingers and cut across using your fingers as a guide to cut a straight line.

CR CR CR CR CR CR CR CR CR CR CR CR CR CR CR CR CR CR CR CR CR CR CR CR CR CR CR

CR

Long Hair "V" Shape Trim

Part your hair in the middle from front to back making two sections of hair. Bring both sections forward over each shoulder. Secure one side in a ponytail to keep it out of the way. Tilt your head back and brush the hair section forward. Using your index and middle finger smooth the hair and hold it place where you want it trimmed. Use your fingers as a guide for the scissors. Repeat with the other side.

CRCRCRCRCRCRCRCRCRCRCRCRCRCRCRCRCRCRCRCRCRCRCR

Long Hair Straight Across Trim

If you don't want a "V" shape in your hair put your hair into a ponytail at the base of your neck and pull the ponytail holder to the end of your hair. Then, clip off the little point.

CRCRCRCRCRCRCRCRCRCRCRCRCRCRCRCRCRCRCRCRCRCRCR

Long Hair Layer Trim

Brush all your hair forward toward your face. Gather the hair and make a ponytail at the top of your forehead with an elastic band. Comb the ponytail to make it smooth. Using your index and middle fingers slide down the ponytail to the desired length. Holding the hair with your fingers trim across with scissors.

CRCRCRCRCRCRCRCRCRCRCRCRCRCRCRCRCRCRCRCRCRCRCR

CUT
&
STYLING

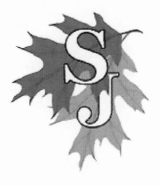

ŒŒŒŒŒŒŒŒŒŒŒŒŒŒŒŒŒŒŒŒŒŒŒŒŒŒŒŒ

Whole Head/Layer Method

Bend over gathering all your hair to the top and center of your head making a ponytail. Rotate and/or twist the ponytail. Trim a half to one inch off. Rotate the ponytail in the opposite direction and trim off any missed pieces of hair. Remove the ponytail. Again with head bent over, run your fingers through your hair to see if there are any pieces that need trimmed.

ŒŒŒŒŒŒŒŒŒŒŒŒŒŒŒŒŒŒŒŒŒŒŒŒŒŒŒŒ

Tip: remember when cutting hair that it is better to cut a little than a lot.

ŒŒŒŒŒŒŒŒŒŒŒŒŒŒŒŒŒŒŒŒŒŒŒŒŒŒŒŒ

Layered Cut

Find your natural part on the top of your head (back to front). Next to this part, create another part about ¼ inch wide parallel with your natural part. Comb this section of hair up and trim the ends. Repeat with another ¼ inch wide section of hair. Always pull the hair straight up. Continue until you have done one side of your part (not the sides) Then go to the other side of the part and do the same thing.

Next, instead of the parts going front to back, you will be doing them from side to side, but only with the section of hair you have already cut. This is to ensure you have trimmed your hair evenly and not missed any hairs. Take a ¼ inch section at a time working from the front of your head to the back of the top of your head.

CR

Find your part again. Beginning at the top of your head make a part ¼ wide down to the top of your ear. If you want long layers pull the hair straight up and even with the previously cut top section of hair. If you want less layering hold it horizontally out to the side of your head. Do one side and then other.

Next, part your hair down the middle from the top of your head to your neck. Then make another part next to it. Pulling the hair straight up use the hair you initially cut on the top of your head as a guide as to how much to trim. Continue making parts and trimming your hair.

CRCRCRCRCRCRCRCRCRCRCRCRCRCRCRCRCRCRCRCRCRCRCRCRCR

ଔଔଔଔଔଔଔଔଔଔଔଔଔଔଔଔଔଔଔଔଔଔଔଔଔଔଔଔଔ

Reference:

Natural Home Remedies for Life http://www.natural-homeremedies-for-life.com/homemade-facial-scrub.html

Womansday:_http://www.womansday.com/style-beauty/beauty-tips-products/natural-beauty#ixzz2IMUVNyqZ

Earth Clinic: http://www.earthclinic.com/Remedies/hair_coloring.html

Reader's Digest: http://www.rd.com/home/6-homemade-dandruff-treatments/4/

Experts Column: http://expertscolumn.com/content/20-home-remedies-get-rid-dandruff-dandruff-treatment-and-cure

EHOW: http://www.ehow.com/how_8182458_make-homemade-eye-primer.html

EHOW: http://www.ehow.com/how_4895500_make-lipoic-acid-skin-lotion.html

EHOW: http://www.ehow.com/way_5763461_homemade-puffy-eye-cream-recipe.html

Livestrong: http://www.livestrong.com/article/27806-homemade-eye-cream-dark-circles/

Care 2: http://www.care2.com/greenliving/15-surprising-uses-for-apples.html

Wellnessmama: http://wellnessmama.com/

Prokerala: http://www.prokerala.com/health/beauty/skin-type-test.php

രു

Medical News Today:
http://www.medicalnewstoday.com/articles/107146.php

Skin Care Resource Center: www.skincareresourcecenter.com

CR

ABOUT THE AUTHOR

Survivor Jane is a preparedness expert, homesteader, and speaker. She is the editor of *www.SurvivorJane.com* one of the world's highest rated preparedness information sites. Survivor Jane is also the founder and creator of the hashtag #PrepperTalk on Twitter, a 24 hour forum that brings people together from all over the world to discuss preparedness thoughts, ideas and suggestions. Jane also moderates the Tweet-Chats on Twitter for National Geographic Channel's hit TV series Doomsday Preppers and Doomsday Castle. Her work has been featured on National Geographic Channel's Doomsday Preppers' BlogTV and website and, many national preparedness blogs and magazines.

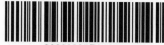

Made in the USA
Charleston, SC
20 February 2014